CREATING COVENANTS

Adrian —

May all you do

heal those you

serve —

[signature]

CREATING COVENANTS

Healing Health Care
in the New Millennium

GLENNA M. CROOKS

Medical Vision Press • Old Lyme, CT

Cover illustration "Workers Building Caduceus" by Dave Cutler used by permission of The Stock Illustration Source, Inc., 16 West 19th Street, New York, NY 10011.

The excerpt on page 80 is taken from "U.S. Senate gets tough on animal activists" by Meridith Wadman. Reprinted by permission from Nature, Volume 399, p. 397, copyright 1999, Macmillan Magazines Ltd.

The excerpt on page 124 is taken from "The care of patients with severe chronic pain in terminal illness" by William T. McGivney and Glenna M. Crooks in the Journal of the American Medical Association, 1984, Vol. 251, no. 9, pp. 1181-1188. Copyrighted 1984, American Medical Association.

Printed on acid-free, 250-year-life paper
Manufactured in the United States of America

To my Father
For my Mother

Contents

Foreword   xi
Preface   xv
Introduction: Breakdown of the Covenant   xxv
Acknowledgments   xxxix

PART 1: FOUNDATIONS OF HEALING
Introduction   1

1. Healing as Divine Gift   3
Stepping into Healing Streams   3
Historical Connections to the Sacred   5
Mysteries of Health and Disease   6
Justice, Retribution, Mischief and Malevolence   7
Wisdom of Divine Law   9
Other Ancient Texts and Practices   10
Hippocratic Mystery and Medicine   11
Christian Mystery and Medicine   12
Secular Healing Traditions   14
Shamanic Mystery and Medicine   17
Modern Mystery and Medicine   19
The Sacred and the Secular: A New Partnership?   21

2. Healing within the Covenant Tradition   23
Covenants: Origins and Meaning   24
Covenants of Grant and Obligation   26
Covenants of Hippocrates and Maimonides   29
The Emergence of Contracts
    within the Medical Covenant   34
Engaging Covenants in Health Care Today   37
The New Covenant among Healers   39
Crafting Covenants between Healers and Patients   44
Reaching Out Toward a Covenant with Communities   46

The Interdependence of Covenants 48

PART 2: MILLENNIUM CHALLENGES AND OPPORTUNITIES
Introduction 53

3. Interdependence: Covenant in Patients' Rights 55
Early Roots of Rights and Responsibilities 55
The Healer's Accountability for Quality 56
The Healer's Accountability for Access and Cost 57
Lack of Reciprocity in the Covenant Relationship 58
Limitations of the Current Covenants of Grant 60
Limitations of Covenants of Grant with Communities 65
Rationale for Covenants of Obligation
    with Patients and Communities 68
The Patients' Bill of Rights 70
Harnessing the Voices of Patient Rights 72
Creating Covenants of Obligation 73

4. Curing Disease: Covenant in the Animal
    Research Conflict 77
Recognizing Needs and Filling Gaps 77
Debating Research 79
Coming to Terms with Animals as Research Subjects 80
Addressing the Tensions and Conflicts 81
Ethical and Moral Views Differ 82
Adaptations to a Changing Society 83
Sophisticated Strategies Emerge 85
Securing Public Support 86
Defending Animal Research 88
Engaging the Covenant 89

5. Making Choices: Covenant in the Tradeoffs between
    Privacy and Efficiency 93
Tradeoffs: Privacy and Confidentiality vs. Efficiency
    and Effectiveness 93
Using Data to Create Efficiency and Effectiveness 95
Privacy Goes Public 97
Involving Patients in the Tradeoff 100
Clarifying the Terms 101
Framing the Covenant to Address the Tradeoff 102
Tough Questions and Dealing with the Details 103
Engaging the Covenant 105

6. Pain and Suffering: Covenant in Conflict with the Law 109

The Extent of Pain in Terminal Illness 109
Addressing Pain: A Critical Test of Covenant 110
Beyond Pain: Suffering 111
Relieving Pain and Easing Suffering 112
Families Seek Better Relief from Pain 113
Healers Respond to Patient Needs 115
Suffering Continues 116
Congress Muddles the Issues 118
Communities in Conflict 119
Confronting the Challenge of Compassion
within the Covenant 120
Creating a Covenant to Relieve the
Pain at the End of Life 121

**7. Healing beyond Our Borders: Covenant and
Medications for the Global Community** 125

Recognizing Need 125
Reaching Out and Responding 126
Healing in the Absence of Explicit Covenants 128
Dealing with Public Relations Disasters 129
Relief on a Massive Scale 131
Seeking a Solution 133
Developing Covenants 134
Managing the Domestic Spin 136
Obligations to the World's Needy Patients 137
Sustaining the New Covenant 141

PART 3: HEALING HEALTH CARE

Introduction 147

8. Emerging Models: Healing within Covenants 149

Practicing in New Covenants 149
Healers and Their Emerging Covenants 151
Cooperative Health Care Clinics:
A Covenant between Patients and Healers 156
Covenants with the Uninsured 158
Celebration Health: A Covenant between
Healers and Communities 160
Engaging Other Healers in
the Community Covenant 162

Reaching Out to the Surrounding Community   164
Reaching Out to Other Communities   165
     ACT Community Outcomes Toolkit   167
Covenant and the Pressing Needs of the Future   168

9. Healing Health Care: Crafting Covenants in the
New Millennium   169
   Coming Full Circle   169
   Only One Step along the Way   172
     Principle Number One: Covenants Flow
       from the Senior Party and Are Preceded by Gifts   172
     Principle Number Two: Covenants Do Not End   173
     Principle Number Three: Covenants
       Change Over Time   174
   Coming into Covenants of Obligation   174
   Who Should Create New Covenants of Obligation?   178
   What Will a Covenant of Obligation Look Like?   180
   Covenants in Action   182
   Evolution of Covenants Over Time   185
   No Easy Answers   186

Epilogue: Questions about Covenants in Health Care   *189*
Notes   *195*
Index   *207*

Foreword

Every now and then a book comes along that is a breath of fresh air. This is such a book. Dr. Glenna Crooks presents a new model for thinking about health care for at least the next hundred years, or, as the title of the book suggests, the entire millennium. Her novel concept of health care as a covenant relationship opens up new possibilities that enable us to escape the fixations and entrapments of the current health care marketplace.

Ironically, the idea of covenant relationships is not a new thought for humanity. It is an old idea and reaches far back into human history. What is new, however, is Dr. Crooks' application of covenant relationships to modern healers, patients and communities.

A covenant, unlike a contract, has a sacred or moral dimension. This is precisely the dimension I find missing in much of health care discussion today, whether that discussion takes place in public policy circles or in the boardrooms of health care institutions. Somehow, legal and business concerns have displaced the more central issues of moral obligation and social consciousness.

Today, there is very little going on in the modern health care arena that inspires anyone. Physicians are dispirited. Many health care organizations totter on the brink of financial disaster. Public health policy is a vacuum. Patients are angry and confused. Third-party payers are targets of public dissatisfaction. Somehow the healing, renewing spirit of the health enterprise has escaped our industry. What Dr. Crooks does so well in this book is lead us through our current labyrinth into the clear light of day.

I hope this book challenges your thinking as it challenged mine. There is simply no easy way out of our present morass. We can't expect a better future by simply doing more of what we are doing now. Increased capital dollars, better reimbursement, renewed consumer efforts, more and better legislation simply won't do it. A new mindset is required that embodies purpose and meaning, spells out mutual obligations and views the healing enterprise as a spiritual calling. This is what Glenna Crooks offers us in this book. Providing health care will always be a business, but it must also be more than a business.

When you read this book, you will have a better sense of the history of the healing enterprise as it developed through the centuries. Better yet, you will gain a vision of how health care could be in our new century. It offers a prescription for a positive future. The author's background in government, public policy and consulting enables her to remain grounded as she explores the reaches of philosophy, ethics, morality and spirituality. For this reason, Dr. Crooks' message is not easy to dismiss. It is not a rambling philosophic essay. It is a focused prescription for building a better health care system.

As a futurist, I am always interested in new visions of health care. I run across many of them. What is usually lacking in these visions is any sense that they could easily become future realities. This is why I am pleased with this book. Dr. Crooks tells us how to manifest her vision. Doctors, patients, hospitals, legislatures, third-party payers and communities must think in terms of the mutual obligations that bind them to one another. These mutual obligations are sacred covenants that transcend single-party interests and rise above simple legal contracts. The covenant mentality is a change of consciousness.

To make the covenant relationship work, everyone is required to make significant changes. Not only providers must change, patients must assume responsibility for their own health behaviors. Patients are as important a part of the healing covenant as the physicians who treat them. We all like to find a single "bad actor" upon whom to blame our system troubles. It is rather sobering to discover there is no single guilty party in the health care marketplace. We have collectively gotten ourselves into this untenable situation, and we must collectively work ourselves out of it. There is bound to be resistance to this discovery. We are quick to point out the need for someone else to reform. We are slower to volunteer ourselves for change. Even communities do not escape covenant responsibilities. They exert a profound effect upon the health or sickness of their members.

I especially enjoyed Chapter 8 where the author reviews people and sites already practicing the new covenants. Patch Adams, Gil Bashe, Griffin Hospital, Cooperative Health Clinic, Celebration Health, Florida Health System, the Accelerating Community Transformation project, and many others lead the way by demonstrating new covenant relationships. Their successes validate the new model. What Dr. Crooks is talking about is not only possible, it is highly desirable.

But before I tell you more about this great book—why don't you read it? Don't skip the Epilogue. It may be the chapter that launches you into a new covenant relationship with physicians, patients and community.

Leland Kaiser, Ph.D.
Brighton, Colorado

Preface

We live in a privileged nation, with abundant resources and opportunities to shape a better health future for all people—not just for those in our own country, but for those in other countries as well. Our discoveries touch the world. Our communications inform the world. Our health care knowledge reaches out to those beyond our borders. Our government is designed to be responsive.

Most people in the world cannot say that. They do not share in the abundance we have come to expect and believe we deserve. They do not have the safe food or sanitary systems that support life, nurture health and enable prosperity. We bemoan the weaknesses of the best health care system in the world by day, and by evening tend our manicured lawns with water safer and more pure than that consumed by most of the world's population.

Yes, we as a nation are not satisfied with the health care services we have. We want more and better care. We demand ever-new advances in research. We are worried about how we will pay for what we receive, and we believe that the prices we pay are too high. We have not taken to the streets in protest, but we have gone to court and to Congress seeking changes in the practice of medicine and the operations of health care businesses. As a result, important policy, political and business decisions are pending as we begin the new millennium. These decisions will shape the future of our own health and that of other nations. The problems we are attempting to solve are just ripening as we enter this millennium. They have been evolving over at least the past 50 years and are maturing with the baby boomers whose aging will stress our creative and financial resources for decades to come. For this reason, it is now imperative that we engage in a thoughtful reconsideration of what we expect from our healers, our healing enterprises and ourselves in the future.

How much of our total personal and national resources will we choose to spend on health care? How will we spend it? How will we allocate our human and financial capital between personal health care interests and societal health concerns? Who will have the greatest influence on those decisions? What role will patients play? Will leadership shift from clinicians and policymakers to patients? Will patients have greater access to information about health and medicine? If so, will they make the right choices as consumers of health care services? What are the "right" choices? Will we as individuals change our lifestyles to support better health, or will we expect medical care to save us from our bad habits? Will we continue to expect society to pay for all of our care, or will we assume a larger share voluntarily, and gladly? Will more of us participate in the public debates in health care to reach real solutions, or will we leave it to lobbyists and Congress to resolve the issues in special interests, polls and partisan political rancor? Will we engage each other in reasoned discussions, or will we make each other the scapegoat for national health care problems?

These questions are directed at those in health care businesses and in the policy, political and regulatory arenas that shape health care markets today. But they are not only for those select few that hold such power. Rather, these are questions for each individual who uses health care services or provides them—for each patient and for each healer. In other words, they are for each of us. These questions are for those who seek care and those who deliver it. These questions are especially pertinent because our founding fathers gave us the gift of freedom, and we, as citizens, have important roles to play within this democracy. We are participants in the politics that are increasingly central to decision-making in health care. These are the questions that will determine our future and that provide the framework for this book.

This book is neither a theoretical text for economists and political scientists, nor is it a treatise for ethicists or theologians. My apologies to each of them if my observations fall short of doing justice to their own analytic disciplines. This book is not intended for academic discourse but for public dialogue—new public dialogue. It is not intended as a scholarly analysis of all the health care issues of the day. That would be impossible. It is, instead, intended as a practical exploration of selected pivotal issues for those interested in understanding the important system changes and public policies of tomorrow's health care. This book is not intended to tinker at the margins of new health care financing proposals or tinker with the margins of health care companies. It is, instead, intended to radically challenge the nature of the relationships that are the foundations of health care today. I will not offer specific solutions or propose changes I believe will "fix" health care—save one. It is my contention that if health care is to be healed, everyone involved in the healing enterprises, from the healers themselves to patients and communities, must enter into new and reinvigorated covenant relationships.

Furthermore, this book is not intended to be a criticism of any individual, organization or political party. There is no need to change the names to protect the innocent because, in my view, there are no guilty parties—or innocent ones, for that matter. Hunting rascals is entertaining, but it is not productive when the goals are healing and change. In addition, creating conflicts is costly and repairing the damage from conflict is even more expensive. As individuals and as groups we have "muddled through" the science and art of healing hand-in-hand with each other and with our national and state governments to arrive where we are today. No individual, regardless of how talented and committed—and I have seen some of the best in action—can undertake the magnitude of all the changes required at all levels and at all times. "It's the *system*." If it is a confused mess, then we are all responsible. We created too many expedient solutions to health care problems and these "solutions" have caused other problems. In Washington, we called that a "bad idea whose time has come." There are too many of these ideas, whose unintended consequences have confronted us with larger problems.

Creating good ideas and making the changes required to shape a positive future in health care must start with the encounters between individual patients and physicians, and so this book addresses the nature of those relationships. Change will take place in community settings, and so it deals with community concerns and imperatives. Change will require the actions of Congress and the White House (as well as state legislatures and governors' offices). Thus, this book also addresses the policy and political tenor of the day. In the new millennium no challenge will have greater immediacy and will reach into the heart of the nation more deeply than health. Yet, as we enter this new era, there are no obvious solutions to these problems, and the political venues for finding solutions are increasingly bankrupt.

There was a time when I thought the solution was in the pursuit of good public policy. If everyone participated in this democracy, I was confident that our collective effort would yield workable solutions to the health care challenges of the day. After all, I had been facilitating public policies in health care for nearly twenty years—as a Reagan administration health policy advisor, as a lobbyist for a Fortune 100 company and as a consultant to health care firms. I have flirted with politics, have been asked to run for Congress and have advised candidates on health care issues. I had no particular training in political science. Like most Americans in these positions—whether in government, in organizations, in think tanks or as activists—I learned about policy and politics by doing. It was not difficult. Policy and politics are embedded in our cultural fabric. They are a part of the national way of life. We teach them to our children, and we encourage their practice in schools and scouts. If "Potomac Fever" could infect my blood, certainly anyone could fall prey to a similar fate. I began my own campaign to spread the disease. I was the "Typhoid Mary" of public policy. I took it everywhere.

I have enjoyed public policy since the bug first bit me in graduate school but began to study it seriously in 1984. I was invited to participate in a meeting among ethicists and academics, government representatives from many nations, theologians from the world's religions and experts from the clinical and scientific disciplines of medicine and public health in Athens, Greece. The group was charged to explore how ethical and religious values affected health policy decisions.[1] My directives as an appointee in the Reagan administration were to describe how health policy decisions were made in the United States and to represent the American experience in case studies of infant mortality, organ transplantation and care of the dying. In preparing for the meeting I began my examination of health policy. It continues and evolves even today.

So, how do we make policy in the United States? What drives our decisions to address a public policy issue? How do we deal with issues? Who makes the decisions? When do they make those decisions? Trade associations, patient disease groups and graduate students came to Washington to learn the ropes and to ask how it was done. My colleagues could explain what legislative button to push and regulatory strings to pull, but I had no simple, clear way to describe policymaking. On visits home, my father would ask, "Now, just what is it that you do in Washington?" I never knew quite where to begin my answer.

Approaching the study of policy the way a sociologist, anthropologist or psychologist approaches the study of a new group, a new culture, or a new patient was useful. What emerged was a deceptively simple paradigm of policy as a consensus-building process with cultural, constitutional and legal roots. This paradigm was embraced readily by my international colleagues at the meeting in Athens—particularly by Europeans—as an accurate representation of their own decision making, and it became a central thread in the conference discussions. In subsequent work in countries around the world, this simple observation has been validated. Along the way, I engaged in a similar study of politics. I saw how conflicts created in politics balanced the consensus developed in policy. The two—policy and politics—danced together. When consensus moved too quickly or too slowly, or when it did not deliver satisfactory results, conflict stimulated the corrective change. Over the long run, policy and politics delivered the goods. They also protected the liberty and freedom desired by the founders of the nation, and that fact was central to understanding the dilemmas of health care. Democracy, after all, was not created to be efficient; it was created to preserve liberty. As a result, pressing problems worsen while political forces balance power and different, but valid, interests. Individual freedoms impede efficient ways to reduce health care costs. In the 1970s and 1980s this meant that health care costs and tobacco-related deaths increased as tobacco farmers, companies and civil libertarians argued for economics of the industry and social rights of smokers. It was not until the late 1990s that slow, incremental steps would make health and the cost of illness preeminent goals. Policy and politics eventually took incremental steps in the right direction. To achieve the desired outcome we needed more—and better—public policies. Or so I thought.

In 1995, believing that public policy was the essential core competency of any important player in health care, I founded Strategic Health Policy International, Inc. Working with clients in all aspects of the health care business—including governments—I continued to see how policy and politics were the domain of every successful company, government agency and health care executive. Through the earliest years of our work we remained optimistic that the policy and political processes that are so embedded in this nation's character would be fully capable of resolving the many issues in modern health care. I believed that conflicts in priorities for research, allocation of health care resources, assurances of quality in care and access to care would all sort themselves out in the policy centers of the nation and the states. I believed that if our clients and all of their stakeholders participated in government policymaking, then collective needs would be identified and successfully addressed—slowly, to be sure, but successfully.

Increasingly, I have come to believe that I was wrong. There are all-too-disturbing trends in health care and government today. Patients are no longer "patient." They are increasingly fearful and feel vulnerable within a system that is intended to be protective and healing. As a result, they are angry and are taking their empowered search for healing to alternative healers and to active politicians. Healers are frustrated as well. Many feel that they cannot provide the care they trained years to provide. At a time when we are on the brink of extraordinary science and clinical practice technologies, healers will be unable to respond to any but the most emergent needs during shorter and shorter office visits, clocked to monitor productivity like some assembly-line factory. Most businesses that comprise health care are engaged in near-term commercial survival tactics, struggling to make investments for the future. Investors are walking away from these formerly profitable operations as regulations and litigation become a greater threat. Policy *analysts* have been replaced by policy *advocates*, who came to Washington in droves to craft the Clinton Administration's health care reform. Single-interest health care *politics* are driving single-interest health care *policies*. Pressures are building to a blowing point. Bad policy created in eleventh-hour, highly politicized debates has become more the rule than the exception.

In addition to understanding how policy and politics—consensus and conflict—work in health care, I began to search for the underlying causes of the anger. I searched for ways to advise clients about how to succeed in an increasingly chaotic market and in such a contentious milieu. My clients were engaging the important dilemmas in health care. At times, the costs of doing "the right thing" seemed insurmountable and the opportunities, nonexistent. I saw good projects and good products fail because the marketplace was too hostile for straight talk, honest relationships and reasoned dialogue. I saw extraordinary discoveries, heroic healing and global philanthropy criticized. I saw dead capital—particularly in human energy and resources—everywhere. The most talented among us could not use the full range of their skills. There was too little time to care for patients, too few funds for researchers investigating viable disease targets and too few leaders willing to risk being the next target of national frustration. Something was horribly wrong.

I believe that the key to dealing with these challenges lies in understanding the breakdown in the healer-patient relationship. This relationship is based on core values of every society in recorded history. When healing was the prerogative of the primitive shaman or village wise woman, and when it was institutionalized by the Greeks who framed our own traditions in medicine, the nature of the healing relationship was that of a *covenant*. Not a contract, a *covenant*. Medical ethicists, in particular William May, Robert Veatch and Edward Pelligrino, had laid the foundation for exploring the notions of covenant. I believed they were onto something.

Covenant defined a relationship, a commitment and an identity for the parties beyond the more common contracts of health care today. Covenant could very well be the seed of the solution. Covenant establishes that a relationship has sacred origins, that no one party benefits to the detriment of the other, that the parties are changed by entering into it and that the parties are mutually interrelated in the venture—as they are in marrying, governing or healing. If notions of covenant were embedded in the earliest relationships between healers and patients, should modern patients expect any less? Would they settle for less? And were they being asked to do that? Could that be the nature of the problem? Have government bureaucrats, third-party payers, corporate providers of health care and even policymakers forgotten that they, too, are healers? Did they ever know that they were healers? Have they broken an ancient and sacred covenant, perhaps without realizing that they are a party to it? Has modern era medicine created so many contracts that we have all lost sight of covenant on the way to the legal department?

Most people today would assert that healers have broken the covenant. Frankly, that is too easy an answer, and it's not true. I am inclined to hold healers accountable, because they are so privileged and powerful—particularly by virtue of the knowledge they have gained through the research and education provided to them, in part, through societal funding. But others are also accountable. Each individual patient and entire communities, as well, are responsible for keeping the covenant. This is only possible, however, if they realize that they, too, are parties to it. In my view, they are. We are all parties to the covenant.

The foundation of the healer-patient relationship was, at the outset, a one-to-one, person-to-person encounter. It quickly evolved into a community-to-community encounter, however, particularly as communities organized to pay for care and healers organized to deliver it. Groups of healers refined their skills, investigated their art and formed guilds. Communities responded by providing healers with privileges and protections. The new, group-to-group relationships mirrored those of the person-to-person dynamics, or should have.

An ancient tribal healer could anticipate that patients would act within the covenant. They would follow the prescribed directives of the healing and would reciprocate the healer's skills and sacrifices with respect for the healing arts. Today's healers can have no such expectation. Ancient communities, particularly the Hebrews, could count on the collective efforts of the group to practice good public health for the benefit of each individual and for the community as a whole. Today's individual patients have no such promise from their community. Healers of millennia past would recognize the limits of healing power, and their patients would do likewise. Today's patients sue for bad results, and courts reach into deep pockets to compensate plaintiffs.

This book will discuss the historical, sacred origins of healing and covenantal roles in more depth. It will begin to unravel the nature of the multiple covenants that exist in our health care relationships today. It will point to a new set of covenants that will recognize more mature, reciprocal relationships. And it will address the toughest question about covenants today: What is the role and responsibility of each player—healers, patients and communities—within the covenant?

Do today's communities of healers—medical associations or corporate providers—act within healing covenants? Will the newly endorsed American Medical Association physicians' union facilitate a return to covenant relationships? Do corporations feel the responsibility to engage in healing as well as in profit? Conversely, do patients and communities heed the advice of their healers? Are patients, who may soon have the right to sue their HMOs, willing to accept their responsibility for the outcomes of their own health? Do communities invest in good public health? Do patients practice good personal health? Do communities assume the responsibility to sustain the healing enterprise with funds and collective resources? Increasingly, the answers to many of these questions are negative.

This is a practical book intended to stimulate a creative, new and positive public discussion to answer those questions. It is for everyone involved in the practice of caring for others and for everyone receiving that care. In other words, it is for all of us. It is intended to end the debate and to begin a dialogue. It is intended to rewire the hard-wired conflicts between people and between communities. It is intended to disarm our hair-triggered willingness to shoot the enemy on the other side of whatever table we share.

It is intended to bring peace to those caught in primal screams and tantrums as they confront the restrictions of managed care—restrictions we collectively and deliberately built into today's practice of medicine. This is a look "back" at the origins of our health care system, and it is a look "forward" to its potential.

Can our health care system change? Can it become a center for the more comprehensive healing that patients now want it to be? Can it be a satisfying place to work? Can it continue to be a vibrant source of new knowledge and life-enhancing discoveries? In my opinion, absolutely! But the potential in health care can only be realized if we cease our endless conflicts and work together. I don't claim to have all the answers to the many pressing questions in health care today and particularly to those related to costs. Costs, in my view, are not the cause of our problems, but in larger part a reflection of them. I do not believe that this book proposes perfect solutions. For too long, the perfect has been the enemy of the good in health care policy. If we can only do good, we will have done better than we might otherwise have done without such an attempt. I do believe, however, that returning to our roots in the sacredness of healing and in the nature of covenants will move us closer to finding more of the right answers. If we do, we will heal not only patients, but also the healers themselves. If we can do that, we will have healed health care. What better time is there than the new millennium?

Introduction

Breakdown of the Covenant

A new millennium provides us with an opportunity to take stock. It is a time to look back and review the past with reflection. It is a time to observe the present with gratitude. It is a time to imagine the future with hope. If we can come to understand the past and the present and not limit ourselves to the health care structures built to "fit" those needs, then we will be more capable of crafting a better health care future for everyone. If we know the paths walked to arrive at today's health care systems, we will be better able to choose to continue walking them or to venture off these paths for new ones. It is likely that after our analysis, we would want to do some of both.

When health care companies and healing professionals prepared for the millennium rollover, they assessed the past, the present and the future. They examined the many choices about what to continue and what to change. They considered the choices that they, their patients, customers or government regulators would most likely be required to make. The principal challenges they identified in this assessment were demographics, technology, demands and resource limits. They observed how the population was aging and how aging people required more health care. They noted that technology was advancing as well. There was not only more of it, but technological solutions were increasingly sophisticated and costly. The public demanded more access to better care. Patients were more informed about their options and more capable than ever of placing demands on the agendas of their employers, providers and legislators. It was recognized that resources were scarce: There never seemed to be enough people, time and capital to meet the needs created by these merging trends.

This dilemma attracted media coverage. The promises of science, the new demands for care, the interests of the elderly and the hostility of patients became front-page news. Health care became good copy. Trial lawyers noticed as well. In the wake of the settlements with the tobacco industry, for instance, litigation loomed as a new tactic to bring the industry to the table—if not to its knees—to force changes in health care delivery practices.

Health care also became good politics. Echoes of stunning failures of catastrophic health care legislation and health care reform faded, but the din from clashes over health care reached Capitol Hill once again—in time for millennium election campaigns. A season of campaign rancor, rascal hunting and eleventh-hour, election-driven political compromises began again. As the nation enters the new century, it risks taking steps away from productive dialogue and toward the demise of a healthy society.

What happened, and how did we arrive at this juncture? How did it occur that healing became such a contentious enterprise? How did the healer's covenant to do all that is possible for the benefit of patients deteriorate? How is it that so many people working for a positive end created so many unintended negative effects? How, even with an infusion of medical expertise into the staff and membership of the Congress, did things seem to get worse even as we knew more? How is it that the United States became such an advanced, industrialized nation with so many of its people—including its working people—uninsured?

Today, all eyes in health care are focused on governments—on both national and state levels—when they are not focused on providers and payers. Was this always the case? If not, should it have been? Is government the right place to resolve the issues of patients' rights and health care benefits? Should the government micromanage health care companies? Are we headed for a crisis, and if so, can it be averted? Many business and policy analysts today focus on the specific elements of the issues in health care: demographics, technology, demands and resource limits. While each of those driving forces of change is important, I believe that it is the relationship between those forces and the players in health care that are the key to understanding and managing the enabling and restraining forces we will encounter in the future. Without delving into the nature of the interrelationships, we cannot appreciate the complexity of the changes that are required to address the challenges of the coming decades.

We face these challenges today for two reasons. First, health care players paid too little attention to government as it emerged as a potent force in national health care planning, management and payment. Second, the traditional covenant between healers and patients broke down—on both sides—and was replaced with contracts. Instead of building on the empowering process of democracy and the solid foundation of covenant, we abandoned both.

Let's begin by addressing the issue of government involvement. To be sure, trade associations and professional societies representing the major providers of health care have traditionally addressed the workings of government at their national meetings, in their association houses of delegates and in the corridors of Congress. But those activities were the turf of a few leadership-inclined members, staff and lobbyists. Usually, they were the policy and political wonks of their own associations—they ran committees and ran for office. National or state policy and politics were an extension of their own personal inclination to be leaders.

For the most part, the practitioners and business executives who were members of health care professional societies and trade associations left policymaking to those individuals while they built their practices and followed their business plans. They appeared in Washington and state capitals only when necessary and contributed to political action committees and campaigns if asked. But for the most part they traded dealings on the Hill for the next deal on the street—whether Main Street or Wall Street. Few of them envisioned a future where the relationship between government and their own health care enterprises would be so contentious as it has become at the turn of the millennium. Such an outcome was difficult to predict in the halcyon days of health care growth.

During the 1950s and 1960s, improving access to health care was the principal driver of national health policy. As a result, the resources available for health care increased substantially. The federal government influenced the health care industry in two critical ways. The Hill Burton Act in the late 1940s built hospital capacity and increased the National Institutes of Health (NIH) budget, which provided more research and research training capacity. In the 1950s and early in the 1960s, institutional budgets grew 15% to 18% annually at a time when the United State's Gross Domestic Product (GDP) grew 5%–9% annually.[1] In the 1970s, Medicare coverage for the elderly and a demand for quality improvements in care increased investments in the health care infrastructure. National expenditures grew from $73.2 billion in 1970 to $247.3 billion in 1980. As a result, health costs emerged as a national public policy issue in the United States in the early 1980s and continued into the 1990s, as the total resources devoted to health care continued to grow at rates exceeding the GDP. Increases ranged from 4.4% to 11.6% annually during the past two decades, always at higher rates than the annual percent change within the GDP.[2]

Because health care was a fast-growing sector of the economy, it was a builder's dream and an entrepreneur's playground. Whether the business was biomedical research, services or bricks and mortar facilities, the opportunities for growth seemed unlimited. Health services employment was a great example of this growth, nearly doubling as it rose from 5.3 million in 1980 to 9.7 million in 1997.[3]

Research and development expenditures in the public and private sectors grew from $12 billion in 1984 to $42 billion in 1995.[4] At the same time, investments in biomedical research were paying off. Of the more than 3,000 prescription pharmaceuticals and 300,000 over-the-counter medicines on the market at the turn of the millennium, most of them were produced since the 1960s. New technologies and pharmacotherapeutics saved lives and improved them. Organ transplants, cardiac bypass surgery and fetal medicine became commonplace. New generations of medicines eliminated side effects and cured diseases that previously went untreated or were managed only through surgical solutions and long periods of convalescence. The polio epidemic and childhood diseases gave way to new vaccines and the appreciation for the prevention of disease.

Not only were health care businesses disengaged from government during this era, patients were largely uninvolved as well. A few politically inclined individuals addressed their special needs through legislation—creating programs for kidney dialysis, rare diseases, transplants and HIV/AIDS—but the average "citizen patient" did not join groups, speak out at town meetings or single-issue campaign to make health care demands. In those decades of growth, patients' needs for access and quality were identified and met without substantial need for broad-based citizen action and coalitions. At the same time, patients became more knowledgeable and insistent about the care they would receive. News stories communicated the miracles of modern medicine and drove demand, while employer-based health care insurance paid the bills for workers and retirees alike. More often than not, patients could count on two things: American medicine would have a solution to their next health problem, and they would be insulated from the cost of the care.

But there were problems looming on the horizon. As the capacity to treat disease improved and demand for treatment grew, so, too, did the population of patients who would require care.[5] Public health improvements and health care services increased the average life span in the United States from 68.2 years in 1950 to 76.1 years in 1996. The population of elderly began to grow at over one million per year, currently representing about 12% of the population and spending nearly one-third of all health care expenditures.[6] Baby boomers started their own families, and birth rates began to rise. As they turned 50, the baby boomers joined the ranks of the "elderly" and became eligible for membership in the first major consumer group with definitive health care interests: the American Association of Retired Persons (AARP). AARP soon became the largest membership organization in the country, representing more than 33 million people over the age of 50.[7] In addition to providing health care products and services, AARP had lobbyists and leaders who were active, engaged spokespersons for many issues—with health care key among them. Employers began offering long-term care insurance policies for workers and their parents. The era of the young-old, the middle-old and the old-old was launched. Centenarians were becoming old news.

Congress attempted to resolve some of the burden for the cost of health care by shifting the risks to managed care organizations. Promoted in the 1980s as a creative solution to the increasing costs of care and the "perverse" incentives in fee-for-service, cost-plus reimbursement, Congress enacted legislation to provide managed care organizations with marketplace opportunities. By the late 1990s, on the heels of managed care's penetration into the private and State Medicaid markets, Congress created Medicare+Choice for seniors in Medicare. This national option for care within the Medicare program soon became a national nightmare. Created in 1997 and implemented in 1998, Medicare+Choice absorbed the unforeseen consequences of a stalemate in a Bipartisan Commission's attempt to save Medicare from insolvency, rising drug costs and anti-managed care sentiment. The Health Care Financing Administration (HCFA) tinkered with Medicare+Choice, creating havoc when it penalized the very efficiencies HMOs were created to achieve. Managed care programs were forced to reconsider their business plans to manage Medicare and by the start of the year 2000, nearly 100 managed care plans that had attempted to serve the Medicare population under this option were in the process of terminating their Medicare plan programs.

In the final decade of the twentieth century, health care had become a payer's nightmare with no end in sight to the problems of unrestrained growth in spending, demand for services and opportunities for treatments. Per capita expenditures for health care rose from $141 in 1960 to $3,759 in 1996,[8] as patients had access to increasingly sophisticated diagnostic technologies and surgical interventions. Employers sought to control their portion of the costs by reducing the share of health bills they would cover, driving some families to insure only the breadwinner, but not the nonworking spouse or children. New ranks of workers joined the ranks of the formerly unemployed and uninsured. These newly uninsured were young workers. Many were employed in information-era companies, small companies and in part-time and nonunion jobs. The ranks of the uninsured grew to more than 40 million and are projected to shoot higher. It was at this time that the health cost control predictions got worse—shots had been fired in the biotechnology and genomic revolutions.

On the eve of the twentieth century, health care was poised to reap the rewards of past decades of investments. But at the same time, tremendous pressures built in health care delivery and financing systems. These issues have captured the attention of the general public, which seems ready to make some collective decisions about what changes are needed. And what will their decision be? Demand more care for more people, at less cost to patients and payers? Demand more accountability from health care providers, especially those profit-making enterprises financed by Wall Street? Health care expenditures had increased over one trillion dollars in a decade, with only a 1%–2% increase in additional healthy, quality years of life for Americans.[9] Something was surely amiss. Providers became "the problem." Controlling providers became "the solution."

On the brink of the twenty-first century, what is the likely future? Beginning in 1993, much to the relief of payers, health care spending leveled out at 13.6% of GDP, and remained there until 1996. The current projection is for spending to increase to 16.6% of the GDP by the year 2007.[10] The aged population will continue to grow. Scientists will become more productive in their discoveries. Consumers will demand more—and better quality—service, but at less cost relative to the intensity of care they receive. Consumers will continue to demand choice, whether or not they are required to pay for it, and especially if they are required to pay for it. Public and private payers will feel the pinch, and it is unlikely that continual cost increases will go unchallenged. Payers will continue to blame managed care, which will in turn blame its suppliers and physician contractors. If history prevails, as managed care companies eliminate utilization controls, additional increases in services and attendant increases in costs will be common. In that event, the idyllic days of growth, consumer satisfaction and unlimited opportunity will be replaced by increasing, unremitting and intractable conflict. Employers will be hit hardest and will pass the blows on to employees. Demanding babyboomers will vote with legislative agendas to secure their rights and will vote with their feet to leave managed care plans that do not meet the demands to do it all—quickly and cheaply. Consumers will pay out of pocket, but only for those alternative and complementary services they value. They will not pay for the traditional clinical care to the degree they can union-negotiate or advocacy-legislate mandatory coverage.

The challenges of the new millennium do not end with the simple need to balance demand and expenditure controls; they are increased by a seismic shift of power and presence among payers and providers. In 1980, private sector payers accounted for 75% of health care expenditures, the federal government accounted for 12% and the states accounted for 13%. In 2000, the states continue to contribute 13% of all health care dollars, but private-payer spending has shrunk to 50% of expenditures and the federal portion has risen proportionately to 37%.[11] One-third of the private market has become public as the health care market share has shifted with the aging population and newly covered groups. As the principal payers of health care, state and federal governments have been forced to become increasingly involved in the regulation of the health care market and increasingly active in seeking public support—through taxes and other means—to meet their responsibilities. President Johnson, in the Medicare debate with the American Medical Association (AMA), reassured physicians that nothing would change in the practice of medicine, except that the government would be paying the bills. As physicians and others have since learned, the power to pay is the power to build or to destroy. Government, as a very powerful buyer, has profound influence over the practice of medicine and the operation of health care businesses. Government is also a regulator of other buyers, acting through tax codes, appropriations, regulations and oversight authority, and, thus, affects the buying of the private sector and even the states. As a result, the federal government is a much bigger influence than its 37% market share implies.

A similar shift occurred for providers. In 1980, physician-driven health care was the norm. Nearly all physicians practiced in solo or group practice arrangements and were responsible for controlling much of health care expenditures. By the end of 1996, 88% of physicians had at least one managed care contract.[12]

Decisions were no longer solely those of the individual practitioner, but often were directed by groups of physicians serving on committees. The committees were charged with directing the practice patterns of those in the group. It mattered little that many physicians continued to practice within their own offices. They were now in contractual relationships with large, business-oriented organizations, which made them responsible for the dual mission of caring for the health of the patient and the health of the corporate bottom line.

Almost imperceptibly, the relationships between healers and patients began to change. There had long been a covenant between healer and patient. That covenant had ancient historical roots and was about to undergo radical change. The nature of the healer and the nature of the patient were no longer the same as when the covenant was established.

George Merck, founder of what is now Merck & Co., said, "Medicine is for the people. It is not for the profits."[13] His corporation adopted a culture in which profit was expected only if the medicines it developed had value to people. As health care companies prospered in the 1980s and 1990s this was a difficult ethic for newcomers to embrace. Investors—not healers—flooded the healing enterprise. Managed care entrepreneurs mastered the art of buying and selling "insured lives," negotiating tough contracts with providers, squeezing the easy, excess capacity out of local health care systems and selling off their companies before the longer-term results would be suffered. They did not build a lasting infrastructure to manage the care. They shook the foundations of care in many communities, leaving a trail of angry patients and providers in their wake.

Even in those health care companies with longer-term visions and health care missions, few people viewed themselves as healers. "Healer" was a term rarely used in the vernacular and, if it was, it was associated with "alternatives" that had little credibility in the maturing business enterprise of health care. Healer might have been perceived as an appropriate term for those in clinical care, but would certainly not have been applied to those who supported the delivery of that care. The growing number of those who worked in health care, but without any direct access to patients, rarely if ever viewed themselves in healing roles. They had fresh MBAs and marketing missions to fulfill, not healing aspirations to accomplish. Those who staffed and managed the corporations providing and paying for health care did not see the connection to the healing of the "covered lives" in their care and their own responsibilities. Insurance clerks, government bureaucrats, congressional staff and others did not engage in covenantal ethics and practice. Patients were too remote from the daily activities of their job descriptions and professional responsibilities. Yet gradually, those who did not even know about—much less ascribe to—a covenant were making important health care decisions.

At the same time, employers paying for health care swept employees into group insurance plans bent on controlling costs. Employers, as paying corporations, negotiated service contracts with provider corporations. Relationships between healers and patients were then increasingly determined by employment contracts. Individual healer prerogatives and patient expectations, demands and rights were no longer central as large bureaucracies began to manage care and money. Some patients suffered as a result, particularly if they lost or changed their jobs and were no longer parties to the negotiated contract. Whether they actually suffered or not, most patients feared they could suffer if these bureaucracies went unchecked. Everyone felt at risk, but for different aspects of health care. Managed care and their physician contractors appeared at risk for costs. Patients feared being at risk for abandonment at a time of need. Corporations feared the risks of increasing premiums and government mandates. Congress feared voter rage from a failure to control managed care and its doctors. Fear had come full circle.

If the increasing health care payment pressures faced by government had not created demands for a renewed political debate, the public certainly would have. In fact, the public was about to do that. More empowered, knowledgeable consumers—many of them middle-class baby boomers who were suffering for the first time from the gap between demand and receipt of health care—started to take matters into their own hands. They held health care providers accountable in the only way they felt they could: They maneuvered onto the health policy and political scene. They demanded change in legislatures and they held government representatives accountable as well, making health care a new, more highly visible issue in electoral politics.

These empowered consumers have arrived and demanded a seat at the negotiating table at a vulnerable time for health care in America. Despite the wealth of opportunity and promises of health care for the future, political rhetoric dominates the debate. Despite the imperative that health care professionals pool their talents and agendas for the good of the nation, selfish interests prevail. Despite the quest for private capital to fund the next generation of technologies and system improvements, regulatory zeal and legislative threats create hostile investment climates. Despite the need for public-private collaboration in areas of research, development and health care services, governments and private concerns view each other with hostility and mistrust. Despite the cry for leadership, few emerge from the limited self-interests of their restrictive economic incentives and personal roles. Those who do are overwhelmed by the immensity of the task of reshaping health care in some rational, but not rationed, way. Is this our future?

Congress addressed the issues more forthrightly than did the professions. Charged with raising the funds and finding new ways to pay for the care—such as requiring employers and the states to pay for some programs—required that Congress engage the public in a discussion of what and how the money would be spent. There were politics, pork barreling and conflicts to be sure, but at least there was a clear, established process to address those conflicts: the policy and political forums at the national and state levels. As campaigns progressed, the candidates touted their plans. Back in Washington and in state capitals, the legislatures debated and voted on proposals. The constituency took note. The press kept score on the evening news.

Health care professionals in the clinical arena were less successful in dealing with these issues. Historically, they had come to feel that they were in competition with each other for limited health care resources. Increasingly, health care professionals lost in those competitive ventures to forces outside health care that grew to control health resources. They did not have a forum to engage patients in a dialogue about the transition to corporate medicine. The relationships of corporate medicine were with corporate America, not with patients who were the employees of those corporations. Employers in corporate America initially acted in the interests of patients and provided generous benefits to attract and retain a workforce. But as health costs grew, the concerns of corporate America shifted. The enhancements to benefit plans institutionalized in the Nixon wage and price freeze era now translated into lower earnings-per-share returns for shareholders and higher costs of goods to customers. Corporations had no choice but to shift some costs of care to employees and some dependent coverage was terminated altogether.

This left the individual healer and individual patient feeling they had little recourse, few alternatives and no influence in their relationships with each other. They certainly, by now, felt they had no covenant. The system may not yet have been broken, but the covenant was crumbling fast. Other players crowded into exam rooms and surgical suites. Peer review and formulary committees, payer clerks, government bureaucrats and investors all had a stake in the process of healing. Some of them actually selected which healer the patient could use. Others controlled which types of diagnostic and healing technologies the healer could use and how often they could use them. Others monitored the encounter after the fact and declared deviations from the norm "fraud." Still others held the healer responsible if the patient failed to follow prescribed advice and did not recover.

The healers, principally physicians, articulated their frustrations the earliest. Some of them, inappropriately, complained to patients during office visits and exams. At times like that, it was difficult to tell who was the patient and who was the healer. Physicians and health care executives needed therapy as much as patients did—not for a physical illness, but for the emotional stress of losing control of their practices. They suffered from the stresses inherent in the growing inability to fulfill the covenant to which they had sworn a sacred oath and were committed personally and professionally. Hospital executives left their positions in record numbers under the stresses. Physicians' economic health took a beating as well, but the uncertainties of contracting were even more significant. Many were left unsure of whether to duck or to run from the next blow. Managed care took a bite out of physician earnings and raised the costs of doing business. Eventually patients complained as well.

Lacking a way to have meaningful discussions to resolve these complaints in the health care, employment or community sectors, each side turned to the government as the only readily available forum to resolve the conflicts. Each of the players was, after all, a citizen of a state and the nation. Whether or not legislatures were inclined to micromanage health care, they were being called upon to do so.

The concerns were popular even when the problems were not clear. The problems were clear even when the solutions were not. Driven by public concerns and political opportunism, legislators embraced the debates with a fury. By the end of the 1990s, legislators introduced over 40,000 health care bills annually into the legislatures across the country. Litigators joined in, too. Patients went to court to pursue their rights to experimental therapies, access to specialist providers and timely access to care for their conditions. Where patients did not have the right to sue corporate health care providers, legislation enabled them to do so. Failing to achieve those rights nationally, attorneys took up the cudgel and sued for-profit HMOs under racketeering theories, hoping to force investors to drive changes in managed care business practices. Not being in the business of forcing social change of this magnitude, investors behaved predictably; they took their risk capital elsewhere and will stay away until the investment climate is more favorable for returns. The managed care sector was thus affected, as was pharmaceuticals in the early Clinton years when investors fled that sector as price controls loomed large and corporate returns seemed at risk.

We enter the twenty-first century with clear challenges and nearly at a point of crisis. The needs of society to educate its youth, rebuild its cities, explore outer space and maintain peace at home and abroad compete with the desires for more and better care of its own health. Employers are no longer a secure source of health coverage and tax-funded Medicare and Medicaid programs no longer provide the safety net of decades past. Future generations have not yet staked their claim in the policy arena and the global internet is creating a whole new set of challenges, opportunities and players in healing and healthcare. These influences are so powerful and moving so fast that it is likely that forces outside, rather than inside, healthcare will have the greatest influence in shaping the future in which the young will live and the older will retire.

This walk down memory lane causes certain pessimism about the future. But it need not. Medical science is poised to reap the benefits of decades of research and deliver on the promises of a biogenetic revolution. New therapeutics will be so stunning in their magnitude that they will challenge the frontiers of our visions about the possible. New practice relationships are emerging between patients and healers, including cash-only practices, pharmacist-led clinical care and entrepreneurs capitalizing on the needs of the nation for diversity and choice. In addition, health care may yet emerge as one of the nation's most recognized assets. Charles Morris, a writer/observer/analyst, offers a contrarian view to those who fear scarcity, by pointing to the abundance of health care today.[14] According to Morris, and I agree with him, health care is a remarkably productive industry. It is a highly scientific, technologic and productive sector. It is a clean, "green" sector, which pays high wages, most of which stay in the United States. Its hospitals and physicians care for people all over the world. Its schools train clinicians for the rest of the world. Its pharmaceutical sector is one of the few remaining industries in the United States with a favorable balance of trade. Its research enterprise is the best on the globe. Busloads of Americans may be crossing the border to take advantage of exchange rates and price controls in other countries to buy the medicines discovered and developed here. But, there are busloads and planeloads of foreign nationals coming here for the diagnostics and therapeutics that are not offered at any price in other countries.

As a society, will we craft twenty-first century health care based on scarcity or on abundance? Will we choose to be generous in our funding of care for ourselves and for the poor? If not, then why not? What are the ethics and values of our nation? How much do we want to spend on the necessities and the luxuries of life? How much do we want to spend on health care? And on which health care goods and services? Will we insulate people from the financial consequences of personal choices that drive health care costs? Will we choose to allow people the personal freedom to engage in health-risky behaviors at the cost of higher health care expenditures? Who will make those decisions, and how will they decide? Which decisions will be made by individuals? Which decisions will be made by physicians and patients, and which will be made by communities, corporations and governments? Which players will be at the table when those decisions are made?

None of these decisions will be easy. A crisis can be averted but only with a substantial change in perspective about the nature of health care. Health care is a personal, one-on-one, intimate relationship between a healer and a patient. Health care is also a collective, public relationship between communities, and between the individual and the community in which he lives, works and travels. Health care is also a covenant that is crumbling before our eyes, but it can be repaired, reinstated and reinvigorated. This can happen within intimate relationships of healing and in public settings. Doing so will require shifting our perspectives. If we can move from contract towards covenant, from fears of scarcity to promises of abundance, from blame shifting to personal responsibility, from rascal hunting to collective problem solving and from conflict to consensus, we might do it. If a new dialogue—not an escalating debate—is created, we can address the more fundamental questions of how we collectively, as a nation, will approach the healing needs and opportunities of the new era.

Acknowledgments

It is a pleasure to recognize so many people who contributed to the conception and birth of these thoughts and words. The first is Edward N. Brandt, Jr., M.D., Ph.D., who, as Assistant Secretary for Health, steered the nation through some tough times in health care during the 1980s era of HIV, Tylenol poisonings and block grants, as well as this junior policy wonk through the transition from Indiana to Washington and global health care. Because of his trust, I had the rarest of opportunities to see leadership from the inside and learn from the best and most thoughtful physician I have ever met. He cared for the nation the way we would all like to be cared for by a healer. Next is Robert Ingram, who recruited me to Merck & Co. in 1988, and P. Roy Vagelos, M.D., who, as Chairman, is likewise trusted. When I first arrived, Roy admitted that he did not understand policy but knew it was important. I think he came to appreciate its value; under his leadership policy attention expanded and gained influence in Merck's business operations. Bob and Roy showed me global business operations in what was the best health care enterprise of its day. Bob brought his own style of covenant commitment to his role in representing the company in Washington and was the very model of covenant-in-action in the policy and political worlds. Like Ed, Roy cared for patients from a distance, but his caring was no less valuable than if he had tended to them personally. He brought them biomedical discoveries and healed millions of patients around the world. My experiences with these gentlemen shaped certain progovernment and proindustry biases that will, no doubt, show through this writing. I say this without apology because my respect for them is well deserved.

I am indebted to an outstanding group of medical ethicists, especially William May. His writings on covenants in health care provide the underpinnings for my own. While our views are somewhat different, I believe they are not inconsistent. We share the same plate of spaghetti—I unravel it a bit differently. He knows ethics and theology; I know health care, policy and politics. I hope he will forgive any less than scholarly treatment of his life's work and will see how his studies have provided a foundation for these extensions into new interpretations of today's health care challenges. As a freshman at Indiana University I was a student of Professor May and enjoyed crossing paths with him again as I pursued the topics here.

I know about politics because Thomas R. Donnelly taught me the live-ammunition, hands-on course and provided the cover when I needed it. I am also grateful to a number of other people. My clients have presented me with their challenges, allowed me to think about their problems and search for policy solutions. Laudy Quintana ran my business so that I could write; Sister Maura O'Donohue, M.D., Sharon Sokoloff, Marty Wasserman, M.D., J.D., Jack Meyer, Ph.D., Malvise Scott, Brian Crawford, Eugene Smith, John Eichert, Carsten Bischoff and Jodie Klein reviewed early drafts and provided helpful reactions and encouragement. Medical Vision Press transformed the idea of a book into the reality with one grand creative stroke after another and provided continued editorial support. The Marisches kept me supplied with surprises during a summer writing sabbatical. The Reverend Patrick McCormick and the Reverend Clif Marquis, ST, provided valuable consultations and comments at critical junctures.

My Dad is no longer alive to see this. Monsignor Joseph W. James was father in his stead—always encouraging, helpful, frequently directing and occasionally demanding. Although he never put pen to paper, he was my writing partner. Mom read the drafts. Of course, she thought they were wonderful—even the versions that weren't. Thanks Mom.

Most important though, I bow to the greatest Healer of all, the Divine Source, recognized by all cultures throughout history as the origin of these healing arts and known by many as the supreme grantor and keeper of covenants. May this work and those who read it reside within the embracing spirit that flows from such an abundant and generous fountain of love and caring. And may health care be healed early in this new millennium.

PART 1
FOUNDATIONS OF HEALING

From the earliest days of human social life, the healers of the community were recognized to be in contact with the most powerful and uncontrollable forces known—those of the divine. The evidence that this was the case is compelling. We know this was true of those ancient groups that left us written records. We know this is true in tribal life today from anthropologists' studies. We intuit this to be true among the ancients who left only their artifacts from the way those items were preserved and arrayed. Healers lived and practiced the healing arts—which were viewed as gifts from the divine—within the context of relationships that were held to high standards of conduct. The material and social rewards for a healer were great. The responsibilities were also immense.

To embrace those relationships and promise the community that the healing practices would be only for the good of the patients, healers followed the example of others in the community who made sacred commitments to one another. These commitments were called covenants. Like the divinely blessed relationships between husbands and wives, fathers and sons, kings and subjects, they adopted a covenant with those they served in their healing roles. Within this covenant, healers called upon their gods to witness their engagement in important, life-supporting arts for the good of each patient, their intent to practice within high standards of technical and ethical care and their wish to be held accountable for their performance.

In those days, the high technology, extraordinary science and complex interplay of today's health care had not yet developed. In these days, we approach unfathomable challenges as biomedical science, health care technology, patient demand and population demographics bring us to the brink of a new era. Into this new millennium we bring with us the covenants created by the first of the healers who sought to care for the patients with whom they had sacred relationships. Many of today's healers practice within the covenants established long ago. More healers should. Covenant is the foundation of all healing practices. Patients expect it and the health of the individual and the community depends on it.

Chapter 1
Healing as Divine Gift

*The government of the United States, under Lyndon Johnson,
proposes to concern itself over the quality of American life. And
this is something very new in the political theory of free nations.
The quality of life has heretofore depended on the quality of the
human beings who gave tone to that life, and they were its priests
and its poets, not its bureaucrats.*[1]

William F. Buckley, Jr.

Stepping into Healing Streams

Angels might have feared to tread into the world of govern-
ment-guaranteed health care. President Lyndon B. Johnson did
not. In 1965, he conceived an extension of President Franklin
Roosevelt's New Deal and called it "The Great Society." It was a
social safety net woven by a government acting as a leveler for the
economic inequities of the day. The Great Society birthed
Medicare and its sibling, Medicaid. These programs formalized
an emerging social contract between people and their government.
It also brought our national and state governments deeper into the
patient-physician relationship in a new way. It used health care to
heal the national disparities in income and the ills of poverty in the
elderly and the disadvantaged. It infused health care systems with
new resources for providing care and, in return, it targeted health
care as a tool for redistributing the incomes of the American people.

The Great Society institutionalized access to health care. It
assured that elderly or poor people (many elderly at that time were
also poor) would receive health care services and would not suffer
from their diseases simply because they were old or economically
vulnerable. It was not the first time that this or any other government
had delved into healing. The U.S. government had cared for its
military in times of peace and war and had provided prepaid
health care for the merchant marine at a time when marine trading

routes were essential to national commercial growth. It had also conducted research and practiced public health.

Other governments and rulers, as recorded in documents as old as the Code of Hammurabi in 1800 BCE, had established hospitals, regulated the healing arts, set its fees and developed medicines. But with Medicare, it was the first time that the U.S. government became a party to the one-on-one healing encounters of its general, civilian population. It was also the first time that American healers were asked, as a group, to balance a national policy objective with the covenant to care for patients. The American Medical Association objected at the time. The result was a political compromise in which the government agreed to subsidize, rather than fully cover, physician fees.

In the end, however, whether paying for all or part of the bills, the government, intentionally or not, stepped into intimate healing encounters. It also stepped into a stream of expectations, relationships, social values and traditions that had been flowing for thousands of years. This stream had swift currents of standard practices, oaths and mores of the profession. It had undertows of theology and ethics that could trap the unwary and uninformed. Healers, whether in the earliest days of Hippocrates or during the legislative era of Medicare and Medicaid, were engaging powerful, magical and sometimes mystical forces. American public policy joined them.

Today, public policy enjoins healers all the more. Federal and state health care programs have grown as populations have aged, as research funds have increasingly flowed from tax-supported sources and as governments themselves, acting as employers and providers, have purchased health care goods and services. The Clinton Administration's proposals for health care reform and universal coverage were spurred by the desires of Americans for more care and their needs for a funding source that would insulate them from the costs of that care. Failed as these proposals were in their government-driven approaches, they were neither the first, nor the last, of government incursions into care. Notably, however, from the outset, American government engaged healers in its public policy agenda without embracing the healer's covenants. The time has come to do so. The time has come to engage others as well— not just government, but patients, communities and corporate providers of health care in today's healing enterprises.

Historical Connections to the Sacred

Scholars suggest in their interpretation of the earliest historical evidence that ancient societies believed they received two gifts from their deity, or from the deities in the case of polytheistic cultures—the law and the healing arts. Whether granted by Isis, Ishtar, Dhanvantari, Asklepios, Apollo, YHWH or a Heavenly Father, both were gifts. Each of these gifts was fundamental to the orderly course and nature of human life. Each structured the nature of community relationships and personal behavior, and each offered a certain security in the face of the harsh unknowns of life. There is ample evidence that this was the case in the origins of the three major monotheistic religions of the more modern eras—Judaism, Christianity and Islam. It is also the case in the major cultures of Asia. It can be inferred for primitive societies by observing the few remaining native, indigenous and aboriginal societies, as well as from the artifacts that some prehistoric societies left behind.

The law provided the vehicle for managing the seemingly uncontrollable behaviors of people in society. Suffer an injury at the hands of your neighbor and there was recourse to a judge to set matters right between you and your neighbor. The healing arts, in contrast, helped manage forces that were more mysterious and uncontrollable than your neighbor. Suffer from an invasion of some unknown spirit or ill humor causing an illness and there was recourse to a healer to set matters straight between you and your god. This was particularly true if it was your god who sent the malady or if your benevolent god was viewed as more powerful than the offending evil cause. Both—the law and the healing arts—were central to the destiny of the individual and the community. Both contributed to the orderliness of society and day-to-day personal and family life.

Powerful legal forces and healing forces emerged in those communities. Rulers and healers were among the most valuable members of society. The sanctity of the social pacts between them and their communities tempered the power they had been given. They were, after all, not only responsible to their people, but to the gods from whom their skills flowed. These pacts were modeled after the covenant experiences of the day. There must have been abuses of legal and ruling power, but the many good kings and judges remain respected in history and lore. Effective healers were legend as well. Sometimes, a single individual like Emperor Vespasian was given both gifts of ruler and healer. He was said to cure blindness, in one case, by anointing the cheeks and eyes of a man with his saliva and in another by allowing a woman to kiss his knee. King Pyrrhus of Epirus was another. He could allegedly heal with his big toe. When his body was cremated after death and the toe did not burn, it was placed in the temple as a holy relic and used for subsequent healing.

Mysteries of Health and Disease

More often, the healers were not the rulers but the priests, priestesses or shamans of the society. In coping with mortality and the more unpredictable and sometimes terrifying forces of health and illness, people sought comfort in the folds of religion. Lacking even the most basic knowledge about the mechanics of the body and unable to even theorize about the nature of genetics, infectious disease and sanitation, their conditions were often shrouded in mystery about cause and effect. As they sought safety from annihilation at the hands of their fellow men under the protection of laws, people likewise sought understanding of the mysteries of life, harmony with their gods, protection from disease and relief from physical pain and death from healers. If a patient died, healers were often called upon to ease the transition to the other world through ritual burial as well. In some societies, as in the case of some Greek traditions, healing was a power not gifted by the gods but stolen from them by man. This made the human healer an even more revered figure. Monetary or some other compensation for healing was granted, but in many societies it was secondary. The real benefit of the healing art was the honor bestowed upon the healer in keeping with the power of delving deep into mysterious forces, confronting them and doing battle with them on behalf of the needy patient.

The intertwining of medicine with mystery and sacred texts is as undeniable as was the rationale. Disease in most societies was associated with either the will of the divine or the work of the devil. In one case, it was the result of both. An entire book common to the Judeo–Christian tradition Bible described the life of sixth-century BCE Job, detailing all manner of physical, psychological and social suffering. This suffering was the result of two mysterious forces beyond the control of this acknowledged upright, seemingly invincible man. One of those forces was demonic, the other divine.

Other texts describe similar forces at play and, unlike Job, recount effective actions to keep the evil forces at bay. In Egypt, it was Sethapop, the great spirit of evil, who caused illness. In Babylon and Assyria, the demon Alu attacked the chest, Labasu caused epilepsy and Nergal was the god of pestilence. In India, Tokman was the cause of fevers. In Persia, six archfiends and thousands of minor demons supported Ahriman, the god of evil. Among the Greeks and Romans, Febris was the god of fever. To this day, our description of illness involving fevers is described as "febrile." In ancient China, families burned bonfires at the edges of property to keep evil spirits and their sicknesses away. In medieval Europe, Pope Clement VI did the same. He sealed himself in his private rooms and surrounded himself with burning fires, seeing no one in an attempt to protect himself from the unknown causes of the plague that ravaged the continent in the fourteenth century. More than half of the clergy of that period died. The pope survived.

Justice, Retribution, Mischief and Malevolence

If not the work of evil spirits, disease might also be seen as the whim of the gods, the result of offended spirits, the malevolence of witches with powers of sorcery and magic. Disease could also be the result of violating God's laws and, therefore, the wages of an individual's sin. King Antiochus, as he lay dying in 164 BCE, attributed his death to his past evil deeds of plundering and pillaging Israelite territory (Maccabees 6:1–13). In modern times, we refer to his belief as "immanent justice reasoning." This immanent justice reasoning has been a prevalent view throughout history. Even Job's friends thought he must have done something wrong to deserve the disasters that befell him.

This view of immanent justice was so strong during the Middle Ages that entertainment was rejected as a form of healing. A group of healers drew upon the recommendations of ancient Greeks to use comedy as a therapy for illness. The approach was much like that of Norman Cousins using Marx Brothers' movies in his own cancer treatment and Dr. Patch Adams using humor in his hospital. Religious groups of the day protested that any entertainment must, of necessity, be the devil's work, as it was the proper place for man to suffer. Try as they might, the promoters of humor and laughter were unable to convince religious healers that a bit of entertainment might help body and soul. Comedy, they reasoned unsuccessfully, might even allow men to return to the rigors of life with a strengthened capacity to defeat evil, sin and the bodily pleasures that destroyed their souls. The religious healers of the Middle Ages ignored the documentation in Proverbs 17:22, "A joyful heart is the health of the body, but a depressed spirit dries up the bones."

Culturally, the church of the Middle Ages, with its practice of canonizing martyrs and saints, sanctified pain and suffering. Illness held a powerful sense of meaning, as is captured in the prayer of seventeenth-century philosopher Blasé Pascal:

Prayer to Ask God for the Good Use of Sickness

Make me fully understand that the ills of the body are nothing else than the punishment and the encompassing symbol for the ills of the soul. O Lord, let them be the remedy, by making me aware, through the pain that I feel, of the pain that I did not feel in my soul, deeply sick though it was and covered with sores. Because, Lord, the greatest sickness is insensibility . . . Let me feel this pain sharply, so that I can make whatever is left of my life a continual penance to wash away the offenses I have committed.[2]

The view of immanent justice was so strong throughout history that it was extended to the sinful condition of mankind generally. Biblical evidence of the suffering required in childbirth, cited in Genesis 3:16, Galatians 4:27, Isaiah 66:7, Isaiah 13:8, Isaiah 21:3–4, Revelation 12:1–2 and Hosea 13:13, indicates that birth was intended to be a painful process as a reminder to women of the "curse of Eve." This view was so predominant that it was used to deny women anesthetic and amnesic drugs, even during difficult deliveries. In fact, it was not until the endorsement of the Lamaze Method of natural childbirth by Pope Pius XII, 100 years after chloroform was first administered to women in labor, that any method to address the pain of childbirth was condoned by the church.

The view of immanent justice was so strong in 1980s America that the HIV/AIDS infection became a major controversy between some religious groups and government efforts to find cures. It is a prevalent view among patients today with chronic pain, and it remains a view held by the educated and elite in the modern era. When asked if contracting a mysterious, serious and deadly illness could be related to evil behaviors of a person, nearly 30% of college students in a recent study agreed that it could.[3] Obviously, the relationship between sin and pain or illness is unrelated to the condition, the era or the education of the believer.

To protect oneself or to reconcile with the gods, the individual required the assistance of higher, more powerful forces. These forces could be engaged with the help of the healer. This was the case in some societies because the gods had granted the healing skill. In other societies, the healers had demonstrated that they

Creating Covenants

could control the divine forces or conquer the evil forces personally. This belief was most pronounced in the shaman tradition, in which the healer traversed the underworld of illness and death and returned to the world of the living. To assure the cure and protect from evil, healers would incant, cajole, pray and employ relics and holy objects. The healer would prescribe prayers in conjunction with herbs, medicines and other therapies and personal, sometimes penitential, rituals. If none of these techniques succeeded in calling forth the gods or in subduing the evil, the priest-healer would invoke the greatest force and mystery of all—the will of the divine.

Wisdom of Divine Law
In Western traditions, formal health care prescriptions and the sacred meet most clearly in Mosaic Law. The ancient Hebrews were no strangers to the power of pestilence and disease. In 1250 BCE they had been saved by their God from the diseases inflicted on the Egyptians who held them in captivity, and they were threatened by Him with a similar fate if they disobeyed Him during their wanderings in the desert following the Exodus. His commands were given directly to Moses, written down and contained in the biblical book of Leviticus. It stands as a remarkable public-health text, with explicit dietary and public health instructions.

Following those instructions was a part of the law that engaged the community's covenant with God, but it was also a prescription for health, disease prevention and longevity. Life was dichotomized into "clean" and "unclean" foods, persons, houses, clothes and utensils. The "clean" could be touched, the "unclean" could not. The "unclean" was segregated from the community, and anyone coming into contact with it required "purification" before they could rejoin society. In characterizing some food as "unclean," requiring ritual cleanliness and limiting food sources, the Hebrews reduced the potential transmitters of disease. Trichinosis was avoided in the prohibition of pork, schistomiasis avoided in the prohibition of seafood. Refraining from touching dead animals, eating dead meat or consuming blood all prevented disease. Inspecting, draining, cleaning and salting meat kept a major protein source safe. Isolating mothers and their newborns following delivery protected both from the harsh realities of ancient life at the time when their mortality risks were the greatest. It assured the growth of the population despite harsh living conditions in hostile climates. Hand washing and avoiding persons with infectious diseases were common practices with the obvious benefits we preach, but rarely practice today. Disinfecting property and clothes to the point of burning dangerous items and vacating homes was also good for the individual's and the public's health.

It was many centuries before public health science would confirm the wisdom of these practices and modern communities would resurrect and promote the simple, clear regulations of this ancient society. Unfortunately, that understanding did not come in time to save a community of European Jews. Because these practices were so effective, there were devastating consequences during the time of the great plagues of Europe. Dr. Balavignus, a Jewish physician, who was cognizant of Old Testament law, the Talmud and the writings of the famous twelfth-century Rabbi and healer Maimonides, recommended to the leadership of the Strasbourg Jewish ghetto that it institute practices similar to those prescribed by Moses. In particular, he advised the cleaning and burning of refuse, and the protection of the water supply from contamination. This reduced the size of the rat population transmitting the plague and reduced mortality in the ghetto to five percent of that of the main Christian city. The survival rate differential was so noticeable, even in the absence of formal public health studies and epidemiology, that the Jews were blamed for the plague and thousands were massacred in retaliation.

Other Ancient Texts and Practices
Even older than Hebrew traditions, Sumerian texts from more than six thousand years ago contain similar references to medicinal gifts from the divine to priests for their use as healers. Buddhist texts of that same period show the relationship between healing and the sacred to be unmistakably clear. In those, Brahma, the First Teacher of the Universe, provided healing information within the Ayurveda, or the Science of Life. This text consisted of 100,000 hymns and all knowledge concerning medicines and healing. The legends describe the gods conquering demonic forces of illness through ritual; through more than 1,000 herbs derived from heaven, earth and water; and through medicines and chants. Disease was seen as the result of sin and, therefore, confession was required. Therapies were effective only when they were combined with prayer and ritual. Buddhist monks and sages passed down the wisdom through an oral tradition, and its current written form, which is still quite extensive and is enjoying a renaissance, is considered to be more limited than the original instructions.

In ancient China, oracle bones were used for divination of the recovery of the patient and then pounded into medicines. Around 2000 BCE, the Second Celestial Emperor developed the national pharmacopoeia by personally testing over 1,000 herbs and 70 poisons—one of which finally killed him. Healing by acupuncture was the gift of the goddesses Scarlet and White to the Yellow Emperor, around 500 BCE. An alchemist Taoist priest, Ko Hung (300 BCE), taught that his elixirs could provide protection from an interesting array of clinical conditions—including ghosts and digestive disorders—and that they could raise the dead and confer immortality.

By 900 BCE the Greeks had institutionalized the gift of medicine from the gods to the point of creating temple hospitals. Apollo was the most powerful god-physician, using epidemics for punishment and healing wounds as rewards. Angry gods caused physical and mental diseases. Appeased gods provided medicines for the favored, especially soldiers. When necessary, the Greek physicians used incantations to secure a healing. Chiron, a centaur, had two famous pupils: Achilles and Asclepius, the son of Apollo. Achilles did not become known as a healer. In one 490 BCE art depiction, he was shown as inept in applying a tourniquet and causing the patient great pain. Nearly invincible himself, he perhaps had no great incentive to be a compassionate healer. Asclepius, in contrast, learned the secrets of medicines to relieve pain. A heavy price was exacted from Asclepius when he ignored the limits to the healing arts imposed on his practice and the risks involved in challenging the gods with too much success. Having committed the unpardonable sin of raising a dead man to life, Asclepius was slain by Apollo with a thunderbolt. Because the serpent and the cock were sacred to Asclepius, they were frequently portrayed with him. One serpent, entwined in Asclepius' walking stick remains the predominate symbol of this healer. In prehistoric times the snake was associated with regeneration, owing to its ability to shed its skin. That practice of using snakes in healing rituals continued for centuries and the image of snakes remains dominant in medical symbols today. Hippocrates, who was born and lived on the Greek island of Cos around 460 to 361 BCE, is said to have stolen the prescriptions of Asclepius before destroying the god's temple, claiming the medicine and snakes as his very own.

Hippocratic Mystery and Medicine

The Hippocratic tradition is rooted in early observational medicine and nearly worshiped today as the beginning of a new, rational era of thought applied to the study of disease. Modern mythology holds that Hippocrates launched the practice of medicine into its current technical and more scientifically-based state. In reality, the Hippocratic practice was actually similar to other spirit-related medical traditions of ancient societies and was by no means free of mystery and magic. Anyone who doubts this connection between Hippocratic medicine and religion need only attend the medical "oath-taking" reenacted for visiting medical VIPs on the island of Cos today. It is an unmistakably religious ceremony, shrouded in ritual and symbol common to religious traditions of the West today.

At the hands of Hippocrates and his students, the cult of Asclepius, complete with snake, spread throughout Greece and to Rome. The god was accompanied by his daughters Hygeia (hygiene), Panacea (cure all) and Telesphorus (convalescence), and his priests built temples of healing where diseases were cured and preventive measures were taught. Everyone who entered the sanctuary of the temples was said to be cured. By 239 BCE, when a pestilence descended on Rome, the locals consulted with the Asclepians at their temple. As they did, a snake emerged from the temple and boarded the Roman ship that had transported the delegation. Believing this to be an omen, the cult became entrenched in Rome, giving way gradually with the emergence of Christianity many hundred years later. We still pay homage, of sorts, to the grand old patriarch of medicine—Asclepius—not with temples but with wallets. To this day, his dominance of healing the sick overshadows the call of his daughters to prevent disease or support caregivers through the convalescence of the patient.

The Greek cults and systems of medicine spread not only to Rome, but also throughout the Arabic world, gradually coming to coexist with Islam. Unlike the emerging Christian traditions in Europe in the same era that addressed mainly the spiritual health of the patient, the Qur'an spoke to both physical and spiritual health. Although the believer was subject to divine aspects of health and illness, there were physical and natural causes of illness as well. A believer was thus advised to bear sufferings for the merits that the trials would bring, but to seek secular healing when the disease became intolerable. The Prophet Muhammad instituted measures much like the public health directives of Moses, and compassionate caring for the sick was a practice of the Prophet himself.

Christian Mystery and Medicine
By all accounts, healing was a significant part of the ministry of

Jesus of Nazareth on whose life the Christian tradition is built. He healed physical and mental conditions. He did not theorize about them; he simply cured them. He denied that illness had anything to do with the sin of the sick person or with the sins of his parents (John 9:1–12). Occasionally He viewed illness as the result of evil spirits, as in a man possessed (Mark 1:23–28, Luke 11:14–20). He believed that there was an evil force loose in the world. This evil was part of a larger picture and illness was only one manifestation of the death it caused. Sickness and death of both the physical and emotional body were part of the realm of the ministry of Jesus and were not intended to end when He departed the earth. Instead, He assigned the closest of His followers with the commission to go forward and, as stated by the Apostle Luke, himself a physician, "cure the sick . . ."(10:9).

Medieval Christianity did not take a step forward in either the science or the art of medicine. Medicine was subordinate to the study of theology. By this time, theology had shifted away from an imitation of the healing practices of Jesus, and now focused on an imitation of His life. Suffering acquired new meaning. The practice of medicine as a secular art, which had emerged in 200 CE with the work of Galen and other scientists, was considered to be inferior to the state of the priesthood. Illness was judged to be either the result of sin or a test of faith. Suffering the trials of pain or disease to gain rewards in heaven was, therefore, the patient's most appropriate response. The love of the healthy body and intellectual curiosity about its functions, which were "givens" within the Greek systems of health care, were not appropriate avenues for salvation of the soul, the more important purpose of life on earth. The dissection of cadavers was forbidden, and the mechanics of the body's inner workings remained mysteries. Healing the patient or curing the disease was not necessarily good, except when that happened by the hand of God or His representatives—especially saints and their relics. In fact, healing could actually interfere with the plans of God for the individual.

Cults of saints were firmly embedded by the Middle Ages, but flourished during this time as their intercession for healing was sought. As practitioners of the healing arts, saints were largely specialists. The image of St. Sebastian, martyred by being shot with arrows, merged with that of Apollo, the archer-healer of the ancient Greeks. The saint was credited with saving Rome from the plague, when in his honor in 680 CE a church was built within Rome's proximity. From that point forward, he became the recourse for the plagues that would all too often and all too suddenly curse the European continent. The word "plague," whose Latin root means "blow, stripe or stroke" of punishment, was, in that case, a fitting term for the meaning attributed to the sudden and widespread illnesses over which the people had little control. The devastation of a plague must certainly have felt like punishment. The hand of St. Theresa of Avila was said to cure jealousy and indigestion. Diluted blood from Thomas of Canterbury cured blindness, insanity, leprosy and deafness. Cosmas and Damian appeared to a physician in a dream to teach him mastectomy procedures. Apollonia—a saint whose teeth were knocked out during her martyrdom—became the patron saint of toothaches. St. Anthony was invoked against erysipelas, or St. Anthony's Fire, as it came to be known in the eleventh century, and numerous cures were ascribed to him. Having a relic in the home, the church and the nation was an indispensable tenet of health care. Saintly body parts were cut up to be dispensed as relics, becoming family heirlooms and talismans against misfortune for the rich and powerful.

Secular Healing Traditions

Although many of the emerging Christian rituals were quite similar to those of the Asclepians, there was a major difference. Christians established a tradition of taking in all patients. Even when non-Christian healers were aligned with a sacred healing tradition, they frequently avoided caring for patients they knew would not recover. They discriminated against the truly ill. A Christian healer ideal emerged out of this practice, and the priest-physician was institutionalized in Europe within the religious communities who cared for the sick. In the Christian community, all the sick were welcome. St. Benedict was one of the early founders within this tradition. He established monasteries that, in addition to other monastic endeavors, cared for the sick. They also grew and studied the various herbs and other prescriptions for treating disease.

During the Middle Ages secular healing practitioners grew in number, coexisting with religious healing for many years, sometimes at odds and at other times in harmony. There is ample evidence that the powerful religious of the day—popes and priests—sought secular remedies. Conversely, secular healers in Europe adopted the formal study of herbal healing as it emerged from the Christian monasteries. Nonetheless, frequently, and especially when the secular healers were women, they were fined, excommunicated, exiled and persecuted as witches using the black arts and invoking Satan in their work.

Secular healers invited retribution from the religious powers because of the patients they treated. This might seem like a conundrum, but it is not. Unlike many other healers throughout recorded history, and even beyond the ethics of the Christians, secular healers were the "healers of last resort" and were less likely to screen out the most critically ill and dying patients. Even the Christian healers who cared for all patients, including the dying, eventually abandoned the care of terminal patients to the providence of God. This was particularly true if patients suffered with pain. The etymology of the term, after all, is derived from the Latin peona, or punishment. Suffering was sanctified by saints and it was sanctifying of souls. As a result, the overriding theological preference for many was to suffer. In the writings of St. Catherine of Sienna, for instance, she describes her choice to suffer on earth rather than in eternity. Death was the last opportunity to assure eternal life, and meddling with the eternity of the soul was theologically incorrect.

It was at this point that patients sought secular village healers for the "alternatives" they offered. These healers took on the cases that others had abandoned as terminal or incurable. Some historians believe that these so-called witch-healers even created their own myths and instilled fear about their potions to frighten away the uninformed, who might otherwise experiment with their powerful herbs—some of which, like digitalis, are still used today. They created this fear by giving common but powerful herbs names that would frighten away the uninitiated and limit experimentation by the uninformed. Digitalis purpurea, a biannual plant with a stem of bell-shaped flowers, is known as Foxglove in our gardens today. It was called "Dead Man's Bells" in the Middle Ages. Other herbals were named "Snake Milk," "Graveyard Dust," and "Beggar's Tick." Only the most foolhardy would dare venture into the "witches'" garden. This blend of fear and respect protected the unwary patient, but endangered the secular healer.

If patients were judged incurable, treated by one of these secular healers and lived, the healer must certainly have touched a power that challenged God's own. As a result, the healer became vulnerable to the political retaliation of the most powerful social institution of the day: the Church, with its ordained healers and its eye on salvation. Once a secular healer emerged in the community, became known and acquired a reputation for success, the healer, and this was usually, but not always, a woman, lived in a dangerous political predicament. Success in healing could bring charges of conspiring with Satan. Deaths in healing, on the other hand, could bring charges of incompetence and murder. Were her "Dead Man's Bells" a tool of the devil to prevent the afflictions sent by God? Or were they used to kill the patient, without benefit of clergy at bedside? Either way, the secular healer was at risk if she had run afoul with the local authorities in the church.

Throughout the ages, healers, with physicians carrying the heaviest burdens, have been held accountable for their failures. This is primarily the reason why some healers took great care in selecting their patients. But practicing without benefit of "license" granted through religious vows carried the most serious consequences of all—regardless of whether the patient lived or died. Hildegard von Bingen, an eleventh-century German abbess whose work in herbals and healing is enjoying a renaissance today, most certainly learned from and taught secular healers of her era. As much as their secular practices were similar to hers, as a vowed religious leader, her practices were ordained as safer and more likely to be in tune with the divine.

Happily, the conflicts were eventually resolved. The Protestant Reformation, particularly Calvin's insistence that salvation come through grace alone rather than through the works (including suffering) of man, separated the body from the grip of the church. Within the church, peace came when all healing, regardless of its nature and regardless of the nature of the healer, was declared to be a "miracle" from God. Furthermore, the church recognized the limitations and frailties of its own religious healers. The powers and prestige of healing and law were abused by some practitioners, and ecclesiastical circles acted in the twelfth century to curb abusive practices by the religious healers. To clip the avaricious wings of its healing angels, several church councils ruled that monks and "canons regular" were no longer allowed to study jurisprudence and medicine for the sake of temporal gain. Financial compensation was banned. The practice of healing and law were not banned, but the financial compensation was.

This was the Middle Ages, several millennia after the first mentions in ancient texts of the sacred gifts of law and medicine. The two essentials of civilized society provided as gifts from God remained squarely and unmistakably in the hands of the priestly class. And, for the first time, the healer class was decreed, by the highest authorities, to provide uncompensated care in their practice of the healing arts.

Shamanic Mystery and Medicine

Anthropological studies of native cultures and their reemergence in modern days confirm the historical interpretations of the sacred aspects of healing in those cultures that left no written records—especially with regard to the shaman tradition. The shaman was a particular type of sacred healer. He, by virtue of heredity or "election," was "called" upon by the community to serve not only in the more secular, herbal healing roles, but in spiritual healing roles as well. The shaman was healer, priest and, when necessary, served as undertaker. He engaged in healing arts, reconciled the soul to the gods and accompanied the soul to the afterlife. It was for this reason that the "calling" was so important. The shaman was the keeper of the collective soul of the community and the healer of the specific souls who sought his care. Initiated into the shaman role through dreams and personal crises of sickness, hardship, and brutal rituals, the shaman experienced the death, dismemberment, and resurrection of his own consciousness. Having come to grips with his own spirits—good and evil—and now in control of them, the shaman was a technician of sacred ways and was able to employ them for the benefit of others. The term "shaman" means literally "he who knows" and it was clear that shamans knew the many mysteries of the forces of power.

The perceived causes of disease and the prescriptions to treat them were similar in the shaman traditions to those groups that we know better through written records. In the Australian aboriginal tribes, the shaman healers use both spiritual and herbal techniques, and are evaluated to assure they can produce miracles. Aztec shamans traced the cause of some diseases and herbal remedies to the rain god Tlaloc. Water-related deaths, such as edema and drowning, were signs that the individual had been chosen to live with Tlaloc in the afterlife. To thwart the god's intentions that the patient join him, the healers employed diuretic herbs to cleanse the body and relieve swellings.

Native North American tribes held similar views and placed the shaman within the priestly class of the culture. Diseases were the result of evil spirits and soul wanderings. Healing occurred through god-given herbs and rituals. Even when, as in some tribes, the rituals were thought by the medicine men themselves to be tricks and "sleight-of-hand" much like our modern-day placebos, they were used ethically and considered effective because the gods sanctioned such tricks for the purpose of restoring health. Like saints in the Middle Ages, native shamans tended to specialize, both in the types of diseases and conditions they would treat, as well as in the types of treatment techniques they would employ.

When European medicine met tribal medicine during the American colonial period, the shamans did not fare well. Both traditions were highly superstitious and neither was far removed from invoking the mysteries of the gods. Nonetheless, early European observers of Native American healing characterized it as uninformed and ineffective. Descriptions by traders, missionaries and captives denigrated both the native practitioners and the patients for practices that were virtually identical to secular and sacred traditions in Europe. Although Europeans believed that "possession" by the devil was a cause of illness, with healing achieved by "casting out" the offending spirit, similar practices among the Native American tribes were discounted as savage. Europeans recognized devils by name and exorcised them. Cherokees, as well, named several dozen spirits, each with a specific ritual for "casting out," but they were viewed as primitive. French Jesuit priests decried the use of charms and totems among the Native American Indians, but mixed water with dust from the tomb of an Iroquois girl, Kateri Tekakwitha, to perform miracles. She was later declared a saint, in part because of those miracles. Native healers remained respected and powerful within their culture despite these attacks, however. In fact, because of their power, they were viewed as a threat to the possibility of assimilation of native groups into white civilization. As a result, early government strategies to transition Native Americans into the mainstream civilization included undermining the respect of the native healer.

Many native healers went underground to survive, to maintain the traditions of the tribal society and to protect the healing covenants they had established with their communities. For example, Christian names gradually replaced the Aztec native names of herbs to protect the healer from being denounced during periods of inquisition. *Peyotl* became "Mary's rose," and *yauhtli*, one of the two principal remedies of Aztec medicine, became "Saint Mary's herb." Old, non-Christian, sacred-origin practices could then continue in safety. Even today, modern Mexican shamans, called *graniceros* or "hail people," make yearly pilgrimages to caves that are swept with "Saint Mary's herb" to assure that evil spirits do not deprive the healers of their powers. Once inside, a blue cross, the symbol of the rain god Tlaloc, is worshiped in a combination of ancient and Christian ceremonies. Just to the north of that region, the U.S. Public Health Service in its medical-care system for Native American tribes accommodates traditional healing practices. Its hospitals include special rooms for important native healing rituals. Medical personnel and native healers practicing among the tribes have reciprocal referral relationships in their practices on reservations. Community Health Centers treating immigrant and native populations with strong tribal-healer traditions incorporate those healing methods and personnel into their base of care and networks of referrals.

Modern Mystery and Medicine

The shaman tradition is reemerging globally, and so are other sacred-method healing approaches. In the 1980s, New Agers adopted shamanic practices in such numbers that Native Americans protested that the proliferation of sweat lodges, ritual dances and spirit healing was a theft of their cultural and religious traditions. While some of those practices might be extreme for most people, the trend to incorporate the sacred into the secular of healing is growing. Even within the most traditional practices of medicine, there is a resurgence of interest in the connection between the sacred and healing arts.

A number of clinicians and scientists are advocates of the connections between the spiritual and healing within the current practices in health care. Some, like Bernie Seigel, M.D., are physicians who have suffered severe illnesses and in the course of their care recognized the relationship of the mysterious and sacred forces to their healing. Others, like Harvard-trained Andrew Weil, M.D., saw the limits of contemporary allopathic medicine in the course of caring for others, particularly when the task was to promote wellness and not just to cure disease.

Some of the connections between the spiritual and modern medicine maintain the mystery of the sacred. Physician and former hospital Chief of Staff Larry Dossey incorporates prayer in traditional clinical practice and is comfortable with "not knowing" exactly how it works. Some of the connections attempt to demystify the sacred, as in Herbert Benson's prescriptions for simple exercises in *Relaxation Response,* or with scientific measures in Doc Childre and Howard Martin's *HeartMath Solution.* Regardless of whether the mystery is penetrated, however, the unknowns and the sacred connections to healing are unmistakably present once again as we care for patients and research disease. Nutrition and wellness expert Dr. Dean Ornish also promotes the value of intimacy. Medical intuitive Carolyn Myss describes the relationship between biography, biology and chakra spiritual centers. Meditation, imagery, art and music—those sources of nourishment typically considered food for the soul—have become medicines for the body as well. Not only have the mind and the body connected in these times, but both have welcomed the soul to the party. Prayer of all sorts is once again present—this time in the healing encounters and enterprises of modern American health care.

A new magazine, *Spirituality and Health,* is on the newsstands. Amazon.com lists over six thousand book titles dealing with healing and a substantial number draw on religion and spirituality as the prescription for the path to health. Weekend healing seminars and tent-meeting opportunities flourish. Faith-based communities offer spiritual and physical healing alternatives, expanding their roles into prevention and primary care, hiring parish nurses and offering immunizations after Sunday services. They also continue to provide institutional care and maintain their missions in the wake of Medicare cut-backs and managed-care competition. Jews, Baptists, Lutherans, Adventists and Catholics merge their spiritual missions with their medical acumen and manage major health care operations. The largest of these is a $40 billion Catholic enterprise comprising 10% of the country's hospitals.

Prayer is not necessarily a subject that lends itself to traditional clinical instruction. Nevertheless, in just the past five years, nearly one-third of the medical schools in the United States have added courses on prayer and healing to their curricula. Prayer is not the common subject of health care administration seminars. But managed-care executives are holding conferences on the subject of prayer in medicine and taking it seriously enough to look ahead to its financial aspects. "Coverage," they state for the record, will depend on "proof that it works."

Proving that it works will take some research, and prayer is not the usual subject of our studies in health care. Yet, researchers are now examining the proper analytic methodologies for investigating its effectiveness. Physicists are hypothesizing the energetic mechanisms responsible for healing through prayer. Ethicists are debating whether prayer should be researched at all. Ronald Kydd in his *Healing Through the Centuries, Models for Understanding* describes six models of miracle-focused healing in which the success rates are within the range of the placebo effects of standard clinical interventions in medicine today.

- In the "confrontational" model, healing is done within the model of Jesus, as a direct confrontation with evil and intervention in the lives of men.

- In the "intercessory" models, those who led exemplary lives on earth and are now saints are called upon to request assistance of God on behalf of the patient.
- In the "reliquarial" model, the remains, possessions or burial places of holy people are the means for healing.
- In the fourth approach, the "incubational" model, patients enter into healing sanctuaries in which they are prayed for over time to achieve the healing.
- In the "revelational" model, God reveals to the healer information to assist in the healing.
- In the "soteriological" model, best exemplified today in the healing ministry of Oral Roberts and most active in the Pentecostal church, God routinely "breaks in" on the lives of men for the purpose of healing and salvation.

None of these models are mutually exclusive, and they are frequently employed in combination. Common to each of these models (with the exception of the incubational) is that the healing will occur instantly. What is useful in Kydd's work is the construction of a language for different healing models that will enable the closer examination of miraculous healing in the modern world. The bulk of miraculous healing is based on self-reports from patients without verification of clinical diagnostics, but then, a portion of our current traditional medicine is based on measures of patient satisfaction that are not dissimilar.

The Sacred and the Secular: A New Partnership?

Whether or not one is religious, honors the sacred or prays, it is undeniable that disease is still frightening and the ordinary terrors of life are still as uncontrollable for us as they were for our ancestors. Healing today may well be even more mysterious. The biogenetics revolution creates even more fear as the causes of disease are not just the external evils of demons or the result of our own weaknesses. Genetics reveals that the uncontrollable ticking bombs of ancestral programming awaits detonation inside of us. In the best of these scientific and clinical times, we may also face the most trying of times in integrating the sacred with the secular in pursuing the public policies for our modern care systems.

On the jacket cover of physician Larry Dossey's latest book, *Prayer Is Good Medicine: How to Reap the Healing Benefits of Prayer*, Ayurvedic physician-guru Deepak Chopra, M.D., says, "With the elegance of simplicity and the precision of science,

Dossey shows us how we can create a lasting partnership between faith and medicine." In *The Scalpel and the Silver Bear,* the first woman Navaho surgeon weaves her fascinating story of transformation from a mechanistic technician trained at one of the elite medical schools to a healer integrating the native with the new. The sacred basis of healing appears to have come full circle and has arrived in modern health care. It will feel at home in the twenty-first century.

Does it feel at home in American government? How strong are these traditions within the minds of patients and healers? How important is this history to the process of healing in a contemporary society? Does this nation feel prepared to abide within the traditions that are at the source of healing and health care and may influence the process of care? Are policymakers prepared to recognize that those who function within the healing enterprise do so within a complex ethical, spiritual foundation? Will public policies accommodate the attitudes and perspectives of these traditions that are harbored so fundamentally within patients? Can a government that stepped into this stream now swim in its waters easily, not only for the elderly and the poor it set out to help, but also for the rest of the nation whose health care it increasingly influences?

A short history of medicine

I have an earache.

2000 BCE	Here, eat this root.
1000 CE	That root is heathen, say this prayer.
1850 CE	That prayer is superstition, drink this potion.
1940 CE	That potion is snake oil, swallow this pill.
1985 CE	That pill is ineffective, consider an implant.
2000 CE	That implant is artificial. Here, eat this genetically engineered root.
2050 CE	That genetically engineered root has harmed other life forms. Here, say this prayer.

Chapter 2

Healing within the Covenant Tradition

The Medicine Trail is a manner of approach, an attitude, like a color of dawn, something that reaches out to touch things any way it can, unformed, created only by the desire to connect.[1]

Stan Rushworth, on Cherokee Healing

Covenants . . . sacredness . . . healing. These are emotionally charged terms. I imagine them echoing through empty hallways in health care enterprises across the country. The halls are empty because everyone has retreated into the recesses of their private offices lining the corridors. I can almost hear them saying, "God forbid that I would be drawn into anything new. I don't have time. Things are tough enough. I have patients to satisfy, budgets to balance and financial losses and premium increases to explain. If it's not the latest accreditation group, quality group or Government Accounting Office (GAO) study group coming to visit, then it's the Inspector General knocking at my door. I've got a business to run—no, a business to save. I've got reporters and trial lawyers looking for trouble. I don't have time for covenants and sacredness in healing."

As health care executives under stress, we naturally reject new ideas that sound like impossible new demands. As Americans, we separate church and state, and these words feel churchlike in a state-focused, if not state-controlled, health care economy. As clinicians, policymakers and payers, we separate soul and science, and words such as "sacred" and "covenant" sound too much like soul in an era that demands scientific application to everything pertaining to health care, including the art of medicine. Besides, for many of us in health care, even our own souls have taken a beating in the course of caring for the nation. Is this what we signed on for years ago when our education began? How can we initiate a dialogue like this? How can we possibly engage in a dialogue like this? How can we give even more of ourselves to patients and communities when all we get in return is hostility? How can we heal others when we are suffering ourselves?

Nonetheless, whether we like it or not, it is undeniable that these "sacred" concepts are rooted in our culture. They are embedded in our language and, like it or not, they frame our debates. Scan the reaction to the recent announcement of the American Medical Association (AMA) that it would support unions for physicians who are employees. Covenant is an implied foundation of these comments. Articles and editorials across the country are outraged that physicians would even consider violating their oath and subliminally remind physicians that they cannot dare to do so. No reporter or editorial writer explicitly connects the oath with its traditions and origins in the sacred or in covenant. No writer needs to do that. The concepts of covenant, oath, sacred and healing are so embedded in our traditions that we take them for granted. They are like the ground on which we walk.

Health, healing, holy, priesthood and sanctuary are inextricably linked in our language. "Heal," "holy" and "sanctuary" arise from the same ancient root word, "hal." The term and its usage grew from life experiences and became entwined in our deepest linguistic origins. These concepts reside within the Judeo–Christian influences that dominate our mainstream culture, and they resonate as well with the Islamic, Buddhist and Hindu views that are increasingly a part of our national consciousness—and certainly a part of our world view. These religious-origin ideas, as different as they may appear in the nature and expression of their theology, come together in their recognition of the sacred within the healing encounter.

Covenants: Origins and Meaning

It was not only the language of healing that grew from the sacred but also the structure and relationships within which healing occurs that grew from the sacred. That structure was provided within covenants. It is unclear in the literature if covenants, as well as healing and law, were viewed as being endowed originally by the divine. What is clear, however, is that "covenants" were employed by God on notable occasions and used for divine purpose— including health and healing. The most notable of these is found in the covenant between God and Moses at Sinai. As a result, the practices of healing developed in communities alongside the emergence and practice of the covenants that structured the patient-healer and community relationships to support the health of

---

Creating Covenants

people. The elements of covenantal relationships and covenantal thought were embedded in the original medical oaths and remain today in oaths and principles of ethical practice.

Both biblical and ancient secular texts are crowded with examples of what covenants were and how societies and covenants developed. Some covenants were between a king and his people, while others were between communities, between fathers and sons, between teachers and apprentices and between husbands and wives. Early Akkadian and Hittite covenants, apparently among the earliest known covenants, established a "covenant formula." Within the formula, covenants contained essential elements. The obligations for a king's vassals, the blessings for obedience and the curses for disobedience were clear. In earlier Hittite covenants, the flow of covenants came not only from the king and carried the force of his law, but the gods of the society witnessed the covenant and were incorporated, by reference, into the agreement. Later, biblical covenants would follow that established rule. These covenants—both ancient and modern—structured the nature of the relationships between the parties in a particular way. We use the term covenant today, but, frankly, we use it carelessly when compared to usage in ancient times from which our current medical ethics grow.

In the context of today's usage, a covenant is:

> an agreement or promise to do or not to do a particular thing; to enter into a formal agreement; to bind oneself in contract; to make a stipulation; a promise incidental to a deed or contract, which is either express or implied; "an agreement, convention, or promise of two or more parties, by deed in writing signed, and delivered, by whichever of the parties pledges himself to the order that something is either done or shall be done or stipulates for the truth of certain facts."[2] [270 P. 2d 276, 278]

Our current usage of the term covenant comes from our current codification of our own laws and distinguishes between several different types of covenants. "Dependent covenants" are those in which the obligation for performance depends upon the actions of another to perform some prior action or meet some condition. "Concurrent covenants" are those in which the performance of one party is required to perform his obligation when the other party is ready to perform his. "Independent or mutual covenants" are those in which performance must be done, without reference to the performance of the other party. Other specifics in the definitions of covenant relate mainly to issues of land, title to land, transfers of land and matter relating to estates. These are not the concepts intended in the use of similar terms in the biblical and ancient texts.

In ancient texts, covenants, by their very nature, involve more fundamental elements of relationships. They are mutual, binding and alter the life and the life-course of any party who enters into them in significant ways. Covenants are typically created between greater and lesser partners—as in a grant of property between a father and son. They reflect the dependency of the weaker party on the stronger party and the superiority of the stronger party over the weaker one. They may or may not bind both parties equally and mutually to a set of expectations, but they are binding and they cannot be reversed. Unlike our modern versions in legal definitions, the performance of one is not dependent on the other, or necessarily concurrent with the other or done in isolation from the other. A covenant, once established, determines the actions of both parties from that point forward, no matter what. And there is more.

In contrast to contracts, covenants are forever. As a result, they transform the identity of the parties. Covenants are not highly detailed. They do not anticipate each of the possible aspects of the relationship over time; to do so within a covenant would not be possible. Because covenants acts within relationships and between ever-changing and evolving parties, the nature of the covenants themselves are moving targets. As the parties to the covenant change, the obligations evolve. In covenants, the giving and receiving is endless and goes deeper over time. The parties to a covenant are continually and mutually responsive and alive within the covenant. Medical ethicist William May said it well:

> A contract has a limited duration, but a religious covenant imposes change on all moments. A mechanic can act under a contract, and then, when not fixing a piston, act without regard to the contract: but a covenantal people acts under covenant while eating, sleeping, working, praying, cheating, healing or blundering.... Initiation into a profession means, in effect, that the physician is a healer when healing and when sleeping, when practicing and when malpracticing.[3]

Covenants of Grant and Obligation

Religious covenants are of two types: "covenants of grant" and "covenants of obligation." These distinctions are important in health care today because of the way in which medical oaths were structured. Understanding medical oaths in the context of these types of covenant points the way to possible solutions to a number of dilemmas we face in health care today.

Covenants of grant describe a unidirectional relationship, in which one party establishes a relationship of giving—a promise, for example, with no requirement that the other party return the favor. This was the type of covenant between the Hebrew God of the Old Testament and Noah. In this covenant of grant, God promises that He will never again destroy the earth by flood. Noah and his family do not promise and are not expected to perform anything in return. Although they are invited to "Be fertile and multiply and fill the earth" (Genesis 9:1), they do not promise to do so, nor are obligations imposed on them to do so. The only promises are made by God. These promises are numerous, and they are significant. And yet, for all the consequences of the promises, Noah is not expected to reciprocate:

> God said to Noah and his sons with him: "See, I am now establishing my covenant with you and your descendants after you and with every living creature that was with you: all the birds, and the various tame and wild animals that were with you and came out of the ark. I will establish my covenant with you, that never again shall all bodily creatures be destroyed by the waters of a flood; there shall not be another flood to devastate the earth." God added: "This is the sign that I am giving for all ages to come, of the covenant between me and you and every living creature with you: I set my bow in the clouds to serve as a sign of the covenant between me and the earth. When I bring clouds over the earth, and the bow appears in the clouds, I will recall the covenant I have made between me and you and all living beings, so that the waters shall never again become as a flood to destroy all mortal beings. As the bow appears in the clouds, I will see it and recall the everlasting covenant that I have established between God and all living beings—all mortal creatures that are on the earth." (Genesis 9:8–17)

This type of covenant of grant is not unlike the one that currently exists between patients and HMO-contracted physicians. Stronger parties—the employer, Medicare and Medicaid, working with the HMO—arrange for physician care for the weaker party, the patient, at the time of an illness. The physician provides a prescription to relieve the symptoms or treat the disease. The weaker party—the patient—is under no obligation whatsoever. He may choose whether or not to arrive at the appointed time for the visit, whether or not to give the physician complete clinical information, consent to diagnostic tests, take the prescription or to abide by the advice given. Like Noah and his family, the patient does not need to promise anything in return.

The second type of covenant is a covenant of obligation. The best-known covenant of obligation in the Western religious world is the one described between Yahweh and the chosen people of Israel. It was to become the central organizing principle of the relationship between God and man, first in the Israelite tradition and, later, in the Christian tradition. This covenant was engaged at Sinai:

> Moses went up to the mountain of God. Then the Lord called to him and said, "Thus shall you say to the house of Jacob; tell the Israelites: You have seen for yourself how I treated the Egyptians and how I bore you up on eagle wings and brought you here to myself. Therefore, if you harken to my voice and keep my covenant, you shall be my special possession, dearer to me than all other people, though all the earth is mine." (Exodus 19:3–5)

The God of Moses grants the covenant, binds the human partners to obligations—to God and to each other—and describes His retributions for their failure to perform. In the chapters of Exodus that follow and throughout the book of Leviticus, the mutual obligations are detailed. The Israelites are instructed on virtually every aspect of their individual, family and community lives. Faithful adherence to those requirements brought territory, prosperity, fertility and special favors. Failure to perform brought punishments, such as the extended stay in the desert that befell the community. Unlike a covenant of grant, a covenant of obligation established reciprocal duties and requirements for each of the parties to the covenant. There was no escaping the covenant. There were no exit clauses. No party could "buy out" the rights, obligations or prerogatives of the other. Thus, care from God was linked to loyalty to God. This relationship with God also spilled over to frame the relationship between men. It was in specifying this covenant that the melding of the sacredness of the healing gifts from the divine become united with the sacredness of the expectations of the covenant between God and man and between men. It was a critical framing of the oath and ethical perspectives of healing and medicine today.

In this biblical covenant, as well as in other covenants, its formation is preceded by the receipt of a gift. According to Professor May,

...gifts precede the promise—just as the gifts of courtship precede a marriage vow, and in the Scripture of Israel, the exodus precedes Mt. Sinai. The Jews bind themselves to God at Mt. Sinai as those who have already received an astonishing gift, the deliverance from Egypt. A covenantal ethic positions human givers in the context of a primordial act of receiving a gift not wholly deserved, which they can only assume gratefully. God tells the Israelites: When you harvest your crops, leave some for the sojourner. For you were once sojourners in Egypt. Givers themselves receive. Benefactors ultimately benefit."[4]

Professor May, in his work with this type of covenant—the covenant of obligation—and its relation to the medical profession, notes that a gift is also present here. Physicians receive an education, which is a gift from predecessors who came before and learned the skills to impart, and from the communities who supported the educational institutions within which the learning occurred. Gifts come to patients as well; they receive the care and healing. The two—physicians and patients—step inside the covenant.

Covenants of Hippocrates and Maimonides
Notions of covenant were reflected in the two best-known ancient medical oaths. The most widely known and used is the Oath of Hippocrates. It is an artful combination of both types of covenants. In this oath, healers, in this case, physicians, enter into a covenant of obligation with fellow members of the profession. They do this by promising to share their knowledge and goods with each other, and to care for each other and their families as if they were one family. They also enter into a separate covenant of grant with patients. In this other type of covenant, they swear to do only good for the patient, protect privacy and confidentiality and practice by ethical principles. The gods witness the covenantal agreement, the terms of which are specified, and the rewards and punishment for failure to perform according to the covenant are invoked:

I swear by Apollo the physician, by Aesculapius, Hygeia and Panacea, and I take to witness all the gods, all the goddesses, to keep according to my ability and my judgement the following Oath:

To consider dear to me as my parents him who taught me this art; to live in common with him and if necessary to share my goods with him; to look upon his children as my own brothers, to teach them this art if they so desire without fee or written promise; to impart to my sons and the sons of the master who taught me the disciples who have enrolled themselves and have agreed to the rules of the profession, but to these alone, the precepts and the instruction. I will prescribe regimen for the good of my patients according to my ability and my judgment and never do harm to anyone. To please no one will I prescribe a deadly drug, nor give advice which may cause his death. Nor will I give a woman a pessary to procure abortion. But I will preserve the purity of my art and my life. I will not cut for stone, leave this operation to be performed by practitioners (specialists in this art). In every house where I come I will enter only for the good of my patients, keeping myself far from all intentional ill-doing and all seduction, and especially from the pleasure of love with women or with men, be they free or slaves. All that may come to my knowledge in the exercise of my profession or outside of my profession or in daily commerce with men, which ought not spread abroad, I will keep secret and will never reveal. If I keep this oath faithfully, may I enjoy my life and practice my art, respected by all men and in all times; but if I swerve from it or violate it, may the reverse be my lot.[5]

Lesser known is the oath crafted by Maimonides in the twelfth century, which he presented in the form of a prayer. Jewish communities viewed medicine as a divine calling. Doctors were given a special protecting angel, and religious authorities directed that a doctor should always be called in time of illness. Unlike others in the community, physicians were allowed to work on the Sabbath, because saving a life was an important task for the community and was blessed by the divine. Maimonides was explicit in his view of how physical and spiritual health was linked. This is a mission statement to which to aspire, even today. Some might say, especially today:

The purpose of the practice of medicine is to teach humanity the causes of ill health, the correct hygiene, the methods of making the body capable of useful labor, how to prolong life and how to avoid disease. It thus directly elevates the human being to a higher moral plane, where the pursuit of Truth is possible and where the happiness of soul is attainable.[6]

The alignment of natural and spiritual concepts is evident in this physician's daily prayer. This is also the first appearance of a covenant of obligation between the physician and patient. Maimonides' prayer calls the patient into a covenant of obligation by requesting that patients have confidence in the physician and his healing art, that they comply with the directions and prescriptions he offers and that they do not take advice from potentially harmful quacks and uninformed family members. Maimonides speaks to a reciprocity in the physician-patient relationship that is ignored by Hippocrates. He steps out beyond the Hippocratic Oath, and its description of the more limited covenant of grant between patients and physicians. Maimonides prays:

All-bountiful! Thou hast formed the human body in Thy complete wisdom. Thou hast united it in ten thousand times ten thousand parts that function continuously to preserve the harmony of the beautiful entity, the mortal integument of the immortals. Ever they are active in complete order, harmony and unity. The moment, however, that frailty of matter or passions disturb this order and disrupt the unity, the forces engage in conflict and the body is reduced to its dust. It is then that Thou sendst to man beneficent messengers, the diseases, who announce to him the danger and urge him to avoid it.

Thy Earth, Thy rivers and Thy mountains are blessed by Thee with healing substances: they can heal. They assuage the suffering of Thy creatures and heal their wounds. Thou hast granted man the wisdom to unravel the secrets of his body, to recognize order and disorder; to draw the substances from their sources, to seek out their forces and to prepare and apply them according to their respective diseases. And Thy eternal foresight has chosen me to watch over the life and health of Thy creatures, and I now go forth to follow my calling. Stand by me All-bountiful, in this great undertaking so that I may succeed, for without Thy aid, man has no success even in the most trivial things.

Inspire me with love for my art and Thy creatures. Do not permit that thirst of grain and greed for fame interfere with my calling, for these are enemies of truth and philanthropy, and they might also lead me astray in the mighty enterprise to further the weal of Thy creatures. Preserve the strength of my body and soul, so that they may be indefatigable at all times to help and to stand by the rich as well as the poor, the good and the bad, the enemy as well as the friend. In the sufferer always let me behold only the human being.

Enlighten my understanding so that I may grasp what is present and correctly surmise what is absent or hidden. Allow it not to sink, so that my judgment may not fail to recognize what is evident but also that it may not overestimate itself and see what cannot be seen. For fine and imperceptible are the boundaries of the

---

great art, and of watching over the life and health of Thy creatures! Let not my intelligence be abstracted. At the bedside, let no extraneous matters rob my spirit of its watchfulness. Let them not disturb in its quiet labors. For great and holy is the search for the preservation of life and health of Thy creatures.

Grant my patients confidence in me and my art, and imbue them with obedience to follow my precepts and directions. Ban from their bedside all quacks and the army of advice-giving relatives and too-wise nurses, for they are a terrible band, who, through their vanity, harm the best intentions of the healing art and frequently cause the death of Thy creatures.

If wiser artists seek to improve and instruct me, let my spirit be thankful and obedient; for great is the field of the art. When, however, conceited fools berate me, then let the love of the art steel my spirit and insist on truth, regardless of age, fame or standing, for to retract in such a case would mean death and disease of Thy creatures.

Grant to my spirit, gentleness and calm, when colleagues, vain of their years, repulse, scorn or sneering try to correct me. Let this also be to my advantage for they know some things that are foreign to me and their self-conceit shall not offend me; they are old and old age is not the master of passions. For I too hope to be old before Thee, All-bountiful!

Grant me contentment in all things, safe in the great art. Permit not the thought to awaken in me: You know enough; but grant me strength, leisure and the urge always to enlarge my accomplishments and to add to others. True art is long, but man's mind penetrates even farther. All-bountiful, Thou in Thy mercy hast chosen me to watch over the life and death of Thy creatures. I now go forth in the pursuit of my calling. Stand by me in this large undertaking, so it may be successful, for sans Thy help man is not successful, be it in the most trifling matter.[7]

The Maimonides prayer is not commonly part of the oath taken by modern physicians, and more modern forms of the Hippocratic Oath have emerged. One such standard revision is:

I do solemnly swear by whatever I hold most sacred, that I will be loyal to the profession of medicine and just and generous to its members. That I will lead my life and practice my art in uprightness and honor. That into whatsoever home I shall enter, it shall be for the good of the sick and the well to the utmost of my power and that I will hold myself aloof from wrong and from corruption and from the tempting of others to vice. That I will exercise my art, solely for the cure of my patients and the prevention of disease and will give no drug nor perform any operation for a criminal purpose, and far less suggest such thing. That whatsoever I shall see or hear of the lives of men and women which is not fitting to be spoken abroad, I shall keep inviolably secret. These things I do promise and in proportion as I am faithful to this oath, may happiness and good repute be ever mine, the opposite if I shall be foresworn.[8]

The Islamic Code of Medical Ethics provides a physician's oath that is similar:

I swear by God the Great; To regard God in carrying out my profession; To protect human life in all stages and under all circumstances, doing my utmost to rescue it from death, malady, pain and anxiety; To keep people's dignity, cover their privacies and lock up their secrets; To be, all the way, an instrument of God's mercy extending my medical care to near and far, virtuous and sinner and friend and enemy; To strive in the pursuit of knowledge and harnessing it for the benefit but not the harm of mankind; to revere my teacher, teach my junior, and be brother to members of the medical profession joined in piety and charity; To live my Faith in private and in public, avoiding whatever blemishes me in the eyes of God, His apostle and my fellow Faithful; And may God be witness to this Oath.[9]

Regardless of the particular form—old or new—the oaths in use in medicine today abide by the elements of covenants established many millennia before. Whether ancient or new, the oaths are witnessed by the gods, and specify the duties of the greater partner (the physician) to the lesser partner (the patient). They create loyalty to their more knowledgable partners (teachers), describe standards of conduct, and invoke rewards and (though less so in modern times) penalties for the quality of the performance.

Did the oaths influence the practice of medicine in those days? It is hard to know. Do oaths influence the practice of medicine today? The Foundation for Medical Excellence, with funding from The Robert Wood Johnson Foundation, studied how oaths and ethical norms governed medical practice in 1997. In results presented at the Institute of Medicine (IOM) in 1998, the investigators noted that there was widespread familiarity with medical oaths, that physicians referred to the oaths frequently, that the oaths influenced their practices (particularly when the physicians were women) and that ethical beliefs and integrity in practice was a critical concern.[10] Another recent phenomenon is also instructive. In 125 of the 145 medical schools in the nation, first year medical students are now "cloaked" in "white coat ceremonies" in which they swear to the Oath of Hippocrates. Columbia Professor Arnold P. Gold, whose leadership resulted in the first of these ceremonies, has noted that taking the oath at the start of medical training is a return to the ancient apprenticeship days of medical education and that it is embraced enthusiastically by students. The ceremony has been promoted as a return to the humanity of medicine at a time when the profession feels its professional values are being assaulted from all sides. It is also an unmistakable return to covenant.

These oaths were historically covenants and remain so today. They are covenants of obligation, but only among the members of the profession of medicine who take them. Unfortunately, patients are not yet a party to any covenant of obligation with their physicians. Furthermore, communities are not called into the covenant in the way that the ancient Hebrews acted as a group to ensure healthy and viable people. The specific duties or obligations of patients are not mentioned, nor are patients threatened or rewarded for their behavior. Patients are not asked or required to take a vow. They do not need to act in any particular way. They will not suffer the consequences of any failure to comply with a physician's orders. The Hippocratic Oath, if it describes a covenant between physicians and patients—and I believe it does—describes a covenant of grant. Is this distinction important? I believe it is.

The Emergence of Contracts within the Medical Covenant
Physicians face a daunting task in the United States to provide clinical care under a Hippocratic-style oath. They practice within both types of covenant simultaneously. The covenant of obligation among members of the profession promotes progress in the healing arts and sciences. It facilitates the development of new knowledge. It also creates a fraternity and provides the support to sustain a difficult life of practice.

But by virtue of the Hippocratic oath, healers also practice within a more limited, and for them, more demanding covenant of grant with patients. Physicians provide, but patients are not expected to reciprocate. There are clearly some returns for physicians that derive from patients—primarily income and respect—but the patient is not, by covenant, engaged in joining the healing venture. Healing is treated as if it was the domain and responsibility of the physician alone, acting within the scope of his knowledge and skill and with the help of the divine. Without the reciprocal obligation of the patient to likewise participate in the healing, it is little wonder that the physician needs to rely on the assistance of the divine. Unlike the values suggested by Maimonides, patients are not enjoined to follow the prescriptions of the physician or to avoid the bad advice of family and friends. If patients were engaged in a covenant of obligation rather than the more limited covenant of grant, they would be more likely to follow directives and assume more personal responsibility for their care. As it is, the physician-patient relationship does not call upon them to do so. To complicate matters for the physician today, the covenant is established with patients, but the process of providing care and the payment for care is established by contract with other parties acting on behalf of the patients' and others' interests. Physicians, acting within covenant, cannot abandon patients. Individual clinicians cannot abandon individual patients, and the profession as a whole cannot turn back several millennia of calendar pages to abandon society.

The emergence of contracts has complicated the demands of healing for any of the healing professions that take, and feel bound by, the covenants as they are intended to function. Contracts are defined as:

> a promise, or set of promises, for breach of which the law gives a remedy, or the performance of which the law in some way recognizes as a duty. [1 Williston, Contracts §1.] The essentials of a valid contract are "parties competent to contract, a proper subject matter, consideration, mutuality of agreement, and mutuality of obligation." [286 N.W. 884, 886]; "a transaction involving two or more individuals whereby each becomes obligated to the other, with reciprocal rights to demand performance of what is promised by each respectively" [282 P. 2d 1984, 1088].[11]

The law specifies several types of contracts. Bilateral contracts are between two parties, cost-plus contracts allow for costs plus a percentage profit, oral contracts require no written documents and output contracts require delivery and receipt of all the products of the work. In contracts, the exact duties and responsibilities of each party are clearly specified and carefully reviewed by attorneys or representatives of the parties. Contracts contain exit clauses and time limits. They limit the rights of the parties in explicitly described ways. Contracts assume at the outset that each of the parties acts solely from self-interest. In that case, it is in the "interest" of one party to guard against the "self-interest" of the other by building in carefully described requirements. Contracts require payment for the expected performance. In contracts, non-performance is anticipated and, therefore, legal enforcement provisions and penalties are built in. Contracts can be enforced in courts.

As a party to a contract with health plans and payers, the physician becomes a contractor. A contractor is defined as "one who is a party to a contract; also one who contracts to do the work for another."[12] A physician is considered to be an independent contractor, or "one who makes an agreement with another to do a piece of work, retaining in himself control of the means, method and manner of producing the result to be accomplished, neither party having the right to terminate the contract at will."[13]

Acting within a covenant, as May has said, requires that a physician live within a "24-7" lifestyle. Being "on covenant" is much more difficult than being "on call" in a physician's practice or "on contract" with a payor. There is no time off from the covenant. There is no time outside the covenant. There is no canceling a covenant. For each of the twenty-four hours of the day and each of the seven days of the week, physicians are bound by the Hippocratic Oath with obligations to fellow healers. They are also bound by grant to their patients. They receive support from fellow healers, but there is no such reciprocity on the part of patients. Regardless of the time of day or particular activity, a healer is a healer—whether in relationship to fellow healers or to patients. Regardless of what the office schedule or managed care contract reads, physicians are always "on call," if you will, in the context of the covenant.

In addition to the parameters of covenants of obligation and grant, today's physicians also practice within the context of a contract. Contracts specify, in greater or lesser detail, how the physician will carry out the covenant. Increasingly, those contracts are specific about how the physician will be expected to practice. Few contracts recognize the comprehensiveness of binding covenant relationships within which physicians are practicing as well, nor could they. As a result, the compensation for performance under the contract is inadequate for the level of responsibility that we expect from these healers as they practice their arts. And then it gets worse. The accelerated introduction of new medicines and technologies places additional demands on physicians working under capitation contracts and living within the covenant. How? Physicians, obligated under covenants to provide for care, must adopt the new technologies they feel are viable for healing patients. Yet, no contract recognizes the increased costs associated with those innovations. As a result, the physician is left in the untenable position of failing to treat for lack of resources, yet living and working constantly within the covenant. The "market" today does not recognize or value that the modern healer/physician lives a demanding, unrelenting, obligation to patients. Is this a realistic or fair and reasonable expectation in today's world? Is it any wonder that physicians, in particular—although they have not been the only healers to feel the tensions of managed care—have bristled under the demands of managed care? Regardless of the circumstances of the contractual relationships, they were still obliged by their covenantal ones. Is the nature of covenant antiquated? Is it out-dated in today's pursuit of health and healing? I think not.

Engaging Covenants in Health Care Today
Although they have ancient roots, notions of covenant and sacred origins of the healing arts are not outdated. They continue to be central to healing enterprises today. This is a critical time to be more explicit about these foundations of healing and return to them in whatever ways possible to address the health care needs of the nation. Doing so will help us come to grips with the challenges and maximize the opportunities in health care today. Failing to do so will stretch our healers to the breaking point and fail to recognize that patients and communities, who heretofore have been passive recipients of healing largesse, must become more engaged in assuring health. Covenants should be central to each of the practices within health care and must be among the fundamental considerations of everyone in healing endeavors. "Everyone" means every individual patient, scientist, clinician, health care executive, government bureaucrat, legislator, and community.

This notion is not new. It was proposed by Dr. Donald Berwick, President of the Institute for Health Care Improvement, and others in a *British Medical Journal* editorial, "An Ethical Code for Everybody in Health Care," published in 1997. In it, Dr. Berwick notes the dilemmas created because important leaders and stake-holders have not adopted ethical codes. This is worse than it might seem, as ethical codes translate into standards and norms of practice. In an informal survey of attitudes he has conducted, for example, 83% of the health care executives responding indicated that a surgeon who develops a new technique to reduce hospital length-of-stay and control post-operative pain is ethically obligated to share his discovery. Only 56% believe that an HMO with similar insights is likewise obligated. Do we really want the corporate healers to abide by different ethical standards?[14]

Everyone should be invited into a covenant—a covenant of obligation, that is. For some, particularly physicians, this will mean re-engaging, re-invigorating and re-inventing the covenants they have held for so long. For others, particularly for patients and communities, this will entail crafting a covenant where no explicit covenant has existed in the past. For still others—those who support clinical care in the health care infrastructure of research, education, management, advertising, legislation and payment bureaucracies—this will require a radical recognition that they, too, work within the same healing enterprise as clinicians, have the same responsibilities to patients and, therefore, should be brought into covenants with each other and with patients. At the heart of crises in health care today is an opportunity to design symmetry and synergy in the relationships between healers and patients, among healers and within communities.

Seeking covenant alone will not resolve all of the issues we must address to achieve the promises of the healing arts and sciences today, but it will help tremendously. A failure to do so will surely contribute to the further decline of the healing enterprise, however, and so embracing covenant in the fullness of its potential should be considered as an important step in advancing the health arts and sciences. A failure to do so will ignore that we can no longer afford business-as-usual tweaks to financing formulas, more burdensome regulations of providers and hand-wringing over patient noncompliance. There are too many diseases to treat, and an aging population is destined to have more of them than ever before. The concept of covenant, itself, is not radical. It is really quite conservative. To recreate and enliven covenants in health care would be restorative and potentially healing for individuals, for the system and society as well. It is precisely the notion of covenant that would enrich health care relationships and allow us to craft the public policy debate on more fruitful ground.

Without such a restorative attempt, we will continue to drift in a direction that strays from its sound origins and is likely to collapse under the weight of its own conflict and confusion. This conflict should be resolved by returning to the foundations of our relationships as healers and patients. This confusion should be addressed by engaging each other in dialogue about what we value within health care and how we will pursue it jointly as patients, healers and communities.

Each of us, at one time or another, participates as a patient in health care today. Even healers become patients, since—as in ancient times—today's healers turn to other healers when they are in need of care. We have the incentive, then, to have an especially close look at the role of patients in the process of healing, including the most important health care measures of all—those practiced by patients between clinical visits, when the critical prevention and treatment regimens are managed at home. Further, we are all, patients and healers alike, members of communities whose decisions about safe water and food, traffic safety enforcement and tax-supported health care will impact on our ability to be healthy.

There is no room in this discussion for old professional jealousies, territoriality, secret incantations of science and mystical methods of clinical discernment. This is a time for entering the heart of the conflicts that drive us apart to find the values that bring us together as individual patients, healers and communities. This should be done by addressing health care covenants at the three levels at which they are broken, weak or unformed: first, among those who are healers; second, between individual healers and patients; third, among those in communities at the local, state, national and even international levels.

The New Covenant among Healers

The model covenants were created for physicians in the Hippocratic Oath and prayer of Maimonides, and it is the physician oaths that are best known. Others in the professions of healing take oaths as well.

Pharmacists swear:

> At this time, I vow to devote my professional life to the service of all humankind through the profession of pharmacy. I will consider the welfare of humanity and relief of suffering my primary concerns. I will apply my knowledge, experience and skills to the best of my ability to assure optimal drug therapy outcomes of the patients I serve. I will keep abreast of developments and maintain professional competence in my profession of pharmacy. I will maintain the highest principles of moral, ethical and legal conduct. I will embrace and advocate change in the profession of pharmacy that improves patient care. I take these vows voluntarily with the full realization of the responsibility with which I am entrusted by the public.

Nurses take the Nightingale Pledge:

I solemnly pledge myself before God and in the presence of this assembly: To pass my life in purity and to practice my profession faithfully; I will abstain from whatever is deleterious and mischievous and will not take or knowingly administer any harmful drug; I will do all in my power to maintain and elevate the standard of my profession and will hold in confidence all personal matters committed to my keeping and all family affairs coming to my knowledge in the practice of my calling; With loyalty will I endeavor to aid the physician in his work, and devote myself to the welfare of those committed to my care.

Associates of the American College of Healthcare Executives pledge to

Abide by its Code of Ethics;
Contribute to the advancement of our profession by exemplifying competence and leadership in healthcare management;
Commit to lifelong learning by maintaining a personal program of continuing education;
Contribute to the improvement of my community's health status;
Enhance our profession through leadership in a wide range of community and professional activities;
Uphold and further the mission of the American College of Healthcare Executives to advance healthcare management excellence.

To engage new covenants with patients and communities, healers today should re-engage their own covenant first. This should be done in several ways. To begin, healers in medicine, nursing and pharmacy with existing oaths should revise and expand their oaths. It is unlikely that, under examination, they will choose to abandon the covenant of obligation that they feel now toward each other. It is likely, however, that they will need to reconsider how those obligations flow to those who are in other related healing professions. For example, it is unlikely that physicians, nurses or pharmacists will decide that they will no longer impart their skills to the younger generation of students, interns and residents learning in the ranks behind them. Even those healers who are uninvolved in formal medical education have the opportunities, and use them, to impart their knowledge to the young.

It is likely, however, that they may consider broadening their view of peer relations to other professional groups who have recently emerged as having particular specialty skills or who have demonstrated the ability to enhance patient healing. Pharmacists come to mind. Recent advanced education, coupled with computer information systems and a plethora of new medicines, have made pharmacists a more important addition to the clinical care team. No longer relegated to counting pills, pharmacists increasingly use their clinical acumen to counsel physicians and patients on appropriate prescribing, dosing and compliance with medicines. As a result, they are no longer subordinate to the prescribing clinician; they are capable clinicians in their own right on whom physicians and patients are heavily dependent. Pharmacists are the only healer today capable of monitoring the increasingly common and potentially deadly practice of patient self-medication with combinations of prescription, over-the-counter and herbal remedies. It would be a missed opportunity for all involved to neglect to marry the professional covenants in such a way that the obligations did not flow freely between the two.

Critical to all the covenants of the healing professions, the elements contained therein should provide the structure for a true covenant of obligation with the patients they serve. It is the stronger party, after all, who creates the relationship and its requirements and invites the other to join. By virtue of the knowledge of the professional and the vulnerability of the patient, it is the professional who must take this first step. This step will involve determining how responsibilities of the patient should be engaged to optimize the healing encounter and support the health of the patient throughout life—on those days when patients are healthy and on those days when they are not.

Having accomplished this task, healers with reinvigorated covenants should lead the dialogue with others in health care that support clinical care and healing. Where necessary, this may mean engaging others in an oath similar to the one offered to health professions' graduates generally. At graduation, some schools offer a more general oath for those entering the healing professions, including those in health administration, public health and management:

> I will devote my professional life to the service of humankind through my chosen profession. I will consider the welfare of humanity and relief of human suffering as my primary concern. I will apply my knowledge, experience, and skills to the best of my ability to assure optimal therapeutic outcomes for the patients I serve. I will keep abreast of developments and maintain professional competency in my profession. I will maintain the highest

principles of moral, ethical, and legal conduct. I will embrace and advocate change in my profession that improves patient care. I take these vows voluntarily with the full realization of the responsibility with which I am entrusted by the public.

Or, if necessary, this may entail developing an oath more specific to the needs of the particular responsibilities of the profession within health care. It is less important whether the oaths in health care are general or specific. It is critical that there are oaths, and that they are pledged and lived by those engaged in healing enterprises today. By everyone, I do mean everyone. On this list, I include without hesitation everyone providing health care products and services for the benefit of people's health. This directs every individual engaged in healing—physician, nurse, technician, scientist, administrator, manager, marketer, insurer, legislator, regulator or government bureaucrat—to become a party to a healer's covenant. This also includes pharmaceutical and medical device companies, e-commerce health care ventures, architects designing health care and living facilities, wholesalers managing the supply chain of goods and telecommunication and financial service companies providing information and financing products. Everyone who participates in or supports healing enterprises is acting as healers did in the past. They are simply doing it in more sophisticated ways and to larger numbers of patients.

Those who now seek to enter the healing arena in the family caregiver, alternative or complimentary areas of practice should be a party to the healing covenant. My mother is healthy and active today, but what happens when she needs more care than her twice-yearly checkups and daily prescriptions, and my brothers and I have to turn to an eldercare consultant, a nursing home, a home-care agency, a physical or speech therapist, a surgeon, a hospital, a hospice and each other for her care? Whose patient will she be? She'll be our Mom, for sure, but she may also become our patient, along with other medical entities and individuals who will help us care for her. Her physician will see her less often and will have less impact on the quality of her life and her health than the rest of us. All of us who care for her, whether we are her children or her home health aides would become parties to the covenant that will care for her. All of us should be willing to embrace the ethics and the values that healers have through the ages, for that is what we will become.

Nobel Peace Prize winner Joseph Rotblat believes that scientists should take an oath similar to that of Hippocrates and vow to do no harm. If it is merely symbolic, he believes that it would lead scientists to consider the ethical and social issues involved in their ventures. I agree. I would add that everyone involved in such a critical area as health care owes patients that same consideration regarding the wider issues.

This covenant of care would extend to those who do not currently see themselves as a part of the healing enterprise. Take, for example, those who watch and report on health care and medical issues. The *Boston Globe* recently announced that in the interest of public health they would no longer run tobacco advertising. They join a small, but growing group of newspaper publishers, including the *New York Times, The Christian Science Monitor,* the *Seattle Times* and the *San Jose Mercury News* who have made similar pledges. Additional steps might now be taken in their reporting and advisory editorial content. A Canadian medical journal study found recently that advice in 50% of medical columns directed at the general public was inappropriate and 28% was dangerous and potentially life-threatening.[15] Similar studies should be undertaken to assess the accuracy of health advice on television network news and talk shows. Beyond the dangerous is the inflated or the incomplete, as well as the unbalanced view. According to a recent study conducted by the National Council on Aging, nearly one in four news stories about research and older women omits critical information. Internet health care providers add to the mix and add greatly to the confusion. Modern patients risk receiving the wrong information, becoming overwhelmed with variously accurate and inaccurate information and becoming underserved by it. Patients lack a solid feel for the real risks to health and are in danger of constantly over- or under-reacting to the evening news and morning magazine shows.

Leaders in health care can make great strides in reclaiming the positions they have lost over the past fifty years by initiating a dialogue to shift the paradigm back from contracts to covenant. These shifts must go beyond the mere mission and vision statements created in corporate climates of medicine. They must reach back to the foundations of care laid down in early civilization and project ahead to the needs of healing today and in the foreseeable future. Those forebears of modern healers may have lacked the scientific basis for their practices, but they had a clearer perspective on the importance of relationship. Therefore, their experiences cannot guide us today in the technical aspects of care, but they were experts in the importance of the climate within which care should be delivered. For whatever they lacked in science, they owned in soul. For whatever we have gained in data, information and knowledge in the past several centuries, we seem to have lost in wisdom. Is it that science has placed such a mountain of information in our path that everything we know is becoming a barrier to treating and healing in ways that are more fundamental, perhaps lower priced, certainly more satisfying and perhaps more effective?

In the early 1980s, former President Jimmy Carter posed just such a question to a group of public-health experts. He posited that we did not solely need more research to improve the health of most Americans. He believed that there was already substantial knowledge that we were not using in the best ways for the benefit of the nation. He wanted to know what could be done with existing knowledge to improve health and how he could best help in any such venture. The deliberations on his question were not easy, because the targets of opportunity were so numerous. In fact, he was right. We already know what we need to know to prevent and treat a vast majority of the diseases in this country and certainly prevent and treat diseases that are most costly. To answer President Carter's question, public health experts assessed disease and risk-factor categories for him. He was advised on conditions such as obesity, smoking, alcoholism and accidents to determine how to change behavior. Should he have looked at the nature of the relationships instead? That is, at covenants? If physicians who know the road to good health and the patients who are asked to walk it day-by-day had better relationships, would behaviors change? Would risks be reduced? Would the results have been more productive if his advisors had approached the underlying nature of the care-giving paradigm? Where would we be today if covenants had been considered in the early 1980s?

Crafting Covenants between Healers and Patients
The model covenants created among healers should then be used to construct a covenant between individual healers and patients. These covenants should be developed initially by groups of healers and patients working together and then modified for the particular practices in health care where they need to be applied. The nature of the relationship and responsibilities of healers and patients within primary care, for example, may be specified somewhat differently than the nature of the relationships in critical care. The ease of access that patients expect for a preventive care visit is different than the access expected for a suspected heart attack or stroke.

Likewise, the healer's expectations vis à vis the patient differ. Healers anticipate that patients will follow the directions for the tablet medicines they prescribe with relative ease. However, caring for a home-infusion drug delivery system is altogether different. Physicians and pharmacists anticipate that patients and families providing for high levels of care will need additional training to assure compliance and proper use. Responsibilities, as well as rights, of each of the parties may vary by the type of care and need to be explicitly recognized.

With model healer-patient covenants in hand, each individual clinical healer should invite each patient into the covenant in a new way, building on the longstanding covenant of grant with patients, and encouraging and even requiring them to participate in a matured covenant of obligation. This covenant would establish the basis for reciprocity and mutual obligation that is so desperately needed now. This reciprocity should go beyond bill paying and social courtesy. Most physicians I know would gladly forego a good restaurant table for a more satisfying practice of the medical arts. It should promote the active participation of patients in the remedies that will promote and restore their health. It would involve those elements of lifestyle and personal responsibility of the patient and their families that would support the continued health of the patient, whether through prevention, treatment, recovery or maintenance activities. Maimonides, for instance, included patients in his covenant, seeking their compliance with his remedies. He also included their families, hoping to protect patients from meddlesome relatives and their bad advice, and warning that their intervention could result in the patient's death. That was a beginning. On that foundation, a paradigm can be built to include patients within a modern covenant of obligation. From the paradigm will come the practices that will, over time, create new insights into the care of individuals and communities.

This dialogue is needed, particularly in an era in which patients' rights and allegations of failures in health care are so prominent in the national policy dialogue. It is the reciprocity of rights and responsibilities of both parties—healer and patient—that must be taken into account. Without defining the relationship—the covenant—in terms that call for patients (as well as healers) to take responsibilities as they secure rights, the goal of achieving health or relieving disease will not occur. Not only is it traditional that the healers initiate this debate, but it is increasingly in their interest to do so. In the absence of such a covenant, healers will continue to bear the burdens of patients' failures to engage in responsible acts. To the degree that the healers and their enterprises are capitated, it is the healer, not the patient, who bears the most immediate and identifiable impact. It is true, patients who do not take their medicines eventually suffer the consequences, but healers paid under capitated contracts suffer as well. This is particularly true if their practice patterns, financial performance and public relations are monitored by quality groups, Wall Street, the press and in the late 1990s, tobacco-settlement-era trial attorneys. Failure to take medications will lead to longer spells of illness and sometimes hospitalizations. Failure to be immunized will do likewise. Failure to eat well, lose weight and exercise will increase the costs of preventive care for hypertension. Inappropriate uses of over-the-counter medicines cause overdoses, accidental poisonings and adverse-event interactions with prescriptions. Self-treatment without learned guidance can cause medical crises.

Respected health policy observer, Eli Ginzberg, reflected on his own experiences when he asked,

> What is the most important lesson I derived . . . over a span of 70 years? Americans think of illness and disability as a condition that can be fixed by an expert, in this case a physician. Accordingly, they want more medicine, more research and more physicians—all with a lower cost and equitable distribution. This was the case in 1930 and it is still the case today at century's end. However, the fact that each individual is ultimately responsible for the maintenance of his or her own health is a lesson that most Americans still need to learn.[16]

Reaching Out Toward a Covenant with Communities

The notions of covenant in healing should extend beyond the person-to-person encounters among physicians and between physicians and patients. Communities themselves are parties to health and should be invited to establish covenant relationships as well. What is a community? A community is a group of employees who work for the same employer; a community is a town, a county, a state. By extension, the United States is a community. In a shrinking globe, with the ready availability of international travel, the internet and ability of people and diseases to travel the globe within a matter of hours, a community extends beyond our borders to include the entire world.

What about the covenants among the members of the community? The most stunning advances in health have been made because of community-level action over the past 100 years. Increasing life span and improvements in the day-to-day quality of life were achieved not by medical care, but by the nearly invisible work and unsung heroes of public health. Modern science traces its understanding of public health back several hundred years. Ancient texts trace public health as far back as the divine edicts of God to Moses. Our living together, sharing common water, shelter, storage and sewage enables our sharing of common plagues and bad habits. Our support of the public health infrastructure is, therefore, critical. Unfortunately, our funding of public health is appalling and our recognition of its importance occurs only when the infrastructure breaks down and diseases break through. Experiences with *E. coli* 0157:H7 contamination of food at state fairs and fast food restaurants, rabies exposure to children at petting farms and West Nile Virus Encephalitis should be enough to raise our awareness of the importance of maintaining the public health infrastructure, even in a very developed nation such as ours.

Public health today means more than just the safety and security of the community's infrastructure. It also includes our personal risk-taking behaviors. We increasingly impinge on the quality of each other's lives. We smoke, abuse alcohol and drugs, carry guns, drive fast, forget seatbelts, neglect immunizations, shun prenatal care and spread sexually transmitted diseases. When these risky behaviors result in high-cost illnesses and disabilities, we burden the tax-based and employer-paid systems that reimburse healers and health care enterprises for our care. Just as the ancient Israelites learned the interdependencies of personal and public health, so must we today. We must extend our understanding to include the reality that all of the health care we receive—especially when it is paid for in whole or in part through third-party mechanisms—is rarely an individual matter. It is all, now, a community matter.

The Fordham Institute for Innovation in Social Policy has reviewed the data of the past quarter century, and concluded that the nation's Social Health Index is declining. The American Dream may be easier to realize, but as a nation we "feel worse." Why? The Institute measures sixteen aspects of social health: infant mortality, child abuse, children in poverty, teen suicide, teen drug abuse, high-school completion, average earnings, health insurance coverage, unemployment, poverty among the elderly, highway deaths due to alcohol, the homicide rate, affordable housing, food-stamp coverage and the gap between the rich and poor.

Ever since the mid-1970s, as the Gross Domestic Product (GDP) has increased, the social well-being index has been falling, and the gap between the GDP and the Social Health Index is widening yearly. We must expect that these factors, which are so integrally related to the conditions within communities, do have an impact on health status and on health care. Particularly for those measures that relate to the health and well-being of children and families, the measures have been declining most markedly in recent years.[17] Unless communities address these and other factors, the pressures on health, health care and health costs will continue to grow.

Communities must create the reciprocal relationships that will support the health of all their members. This is perhaps one of the most pressing needs in health care today. Not only do we have individual, private and confidential matters concerning our own personal and separate health care needs, we also have needs in common with others. The community is the setting in which our needs and those of others are placed in conflict and can be brought into harmony. Increasingly, our communities have neglected this aspect of collective life. Some of our most contentious public policy issues arise from the collective relationships of community, and some of the greatest potential for resolution lie there as well. Some of the most important ways to improve health and reduce health care costs are born within communities. Smoking, food safety, gun control, traffic safety, immunizations, clean air and water, hazardous waste, rabies in urban animals and pest infestation are community, not just personal health, concerns. Yet, resolving each will require larger budgets and less liberty—tough issues for any community. Addressing these tensions will be one of the essential challenges of the next generation. Resolving them will require that the other covenants are acknowledged, in place, and practiced, if we are to address the critical challenges that an aging population, advances in medical technology and patient demand place upon us. Fortunately, a number of communities are leading the way in models that define health in terms that satisfy their needs and that address the social, economic, behavioral, public health and clinical care imperatives of meeting those needs.

The Interdependence of Covenants
These new, modern covenants of obligation extend the reciprocity in the relationships in a number of ways. They extend the covenant of obligation among physicians to include obligations among all healers, between individual healers and patients and among mem-

bers of a community. They establish obligations of patients for the first time. They reach out to communities in a new way and call on them to be accountable. They create the foundation on which a new dialogue can be engaged in between healers and patients within a community, a state, a nation and around the world. The healing enterprise today, now more than ever, depends on the actions of interdependent parties, acting in reciprocity in the context of a covenant of obligation.

As they currently stand, the relationships between healers and patients rest on the patient's dependency on the physician. This is a role patients have been encouraged to assume. Employers and health care financing systems have facilitated that dependency. In recent years, that dependency has shifted from a clinical dependency on physicians (with financial support from third parties) to clinical and financial dependency on the managed-care organizations that contract with those physicians. Dependency, however, evokes a parent-child paradigm that is wholly unsatisfactory for the fulfillment of health goals and the development of mature health systems today.[18] Remaining childlike in the approach to our own health and healing deprives us of the opportunity to grow towards a greater potential that accepting responsibility entails.

This growth process may be painful. Change and growth frequently are. Without a deliberate covenant dialogue, however, we risk taking steps towards change that will be unproductive. We all remember adolescence and the developmental imperative of that stage of life to assert independence. Today's relationships in health care are taking on the appearance of the familiar rebellions of an adolescent stage of life. In many ways, patients are becoming independent. We are not taking our prescription medicines, are ignoring the advice of physicians and turning to alternatives on our own initiative. It is projected that nearly half the population is now using alternative and complementary therapies and that visits for alternative therapies exceed visits for primary care. Counting visits and the costs of products, Americans spent over $30 billion in 1997, paying for it mostly out-of-pocket. We are combining the prescription and the over-the-counter medicines in ways that may be harmful. We are venturing into the land of herbals and unregulated, unproven products as if the "natural" is always better than today's health care offerings. We're not reading labels and may be mishandling many of the medicines we take. We trust the anonymous sources on the global internet more than the trained and licensed practitioner in the neighborhood. This type of rebellion may, in fact, be a necessary phase of development in human growth. It would be an unfortunate place for health care systems to get stuck, however. The same foundations of science and education that support traditional, clinical care should support self-care, alternative and complementary medicine as well. If managed care today required patients to use these alternatives without the benefit of the Food and Drug Administration (FDA) or other regulatory agencies' assurances of their safety and efficacy, we, as patients, would object.

Neither dependence nor independence is an attractive or satisfying state for adults. Baby-boomers are poised to use their political power to demand more from health care, and they should. They should make those demands with the awareness of their responsibilities, however. The parents of the baby boomers were given entitlement reassurances through Medicare and employer-based reassurances through health insurance. Both created dependencies on modern health systems that are not capable of meeting the demands that the increasingly vocal and powerful elderly population will become as baby-boomers age. With luck and some hard work, especially on the part of the health care community, we may be able to weather the storms of rebellion of this adolescent period in our national patient-driven growth. With policy and political restraint on the part of the legislatures, we might succeed in reaching adulthood without institutionalizing the dependence and independence that is most common today.

The aim for individuals, as well as for society, should be to progress toward "interdependence." If healers, particularly physicians, wish to resume the effective and powerful roles that are deeply embedded in our tradition and culture, they must make the first moves toward creating and offering new covenants. They have both the historical and the legal prerogatives to do so. They remain, by law and tradition, the more responsible of the partners—both among healers and with patients. They should initiate the dialogue with each of the other parties involved in the healing enterprise. They must provide leadership.

When physicians have succeeded in creating a broader group of healers who have adopted and developed practices within covenants, they can then approach the tasks of dealing with patients as individuals and in community. In much the same way that good parents help their children to grow up, the healers of our society should take the initiative to confront the dependencies that they and their forebears have created in the patients they treat.

This applies not only to those healers who are directly engaged in patient care, but also to those healers who are supporting and peripheral in medical care—including those in public health, health care company management, research or public policy. The inclination of all these healers today has been to take too much responsibility from the shoulders of patients and place it on their own.

As a result of assuming all the responsibility and shielding patients and communities from difficult choices, the health care enterprise today finds itself in constant turmoil. It bears the internal conflicts over the allocation of power and professional practice. It struggles with how best to allocate the scarce resources given to it by the community. Its own identity is in crisis as it is being reformed by forces from the outside. It faces controversy with patients and the broader community on every front. Its costs are too high, its quality too low. More and more of its patients, estimates of upwards of 47 million at last count, do not have health insurance. It has become responsible for limiting access and is being sued for succeeding in that responsibility. Its new products and services are perceived as too expensive. Its most valuable practices are second-guessed and underpaid. It is a target of fraud investigations by the Inspector General, the Justice Department and the FBI. Its patients are not satisfied, its healers are not satisfied.

These are crises, but they are also opportunities. It is the opportunities that are the most exciting. We know that much of disease is lifestyle-caused and that a change in lifestyle can improve health. We know we can relieve substantial illness, injury, cost and suffering through the application of new treatment and care paradigms that create behavior change. We know that we can effect the clinical course of certain diseases by changing patient and family dynamics. We know that working with patients within the healing context can save lives. We are learning that the status and involvement of the patient in healing will differentially determine the adhesion of the drugs we prescribe to heal them. We know that communities that support the health of their citizens can enjoy better quality of personal and collective life. Whether we are pushed by threats or pulled by opportunities into covenants, it is the next worthy trip to take.

Part 2
MILLENNIUM CHALLENGES AND OPPORTUNITIES

The new century arrives bearing gifts of challenges and crises. These will provide us with the opportunity to examine how we live our lives, value our freedoms, express our compassion, resolve our conflicts, accept our responsibilities, care for our dying and allocate our resources. These challenges and opportunities will require that we address our immediate concerns for health and healing while we value the different cultural, ethical, social and political perspectives of heterogeneous communities.

How we care for the youngest, oldest and weakest among us will be a reflection of our character. In the future, whether or not we decide to invest in biomedical research, patient-centered care, new communications and the internet, infrastructure development and public health will show how visionary our instincts are compared with those who came before us. How we reach out to the rest of the world with our health care technologies, or whether we reach out at all, will evidence our degree of health isolationism and interests in the global community. How we study our genes, meet the demands of an aging society and balance rights and responsibilities will demonstrate the degree of maturity we attribute to patients and healers. How we monitor and manage the work of healers will indicate how much we continue to trust that the covenants to which they ascribe are active influences in the practice of medicine and the healing arts.

These challenges and crises are gifts, because they will push the limits of defining ourselves as human beings, as members of communities and as participants in healing. These challenges and opportunities will force us to examine each other and ourselves at the depths of who we are and what we view as important. Each can prompt a rich dialogue and can lead us to new, creative solutions to seemingly impossible dilemmas; especially, I believe, if these challenges and crises are examined in the context of the gifts of healing and in the presence of covenants of care.

Chapter 3

Interdependence

Covenant in Patients' Rights

> *Historically, governments that provide rich legal rights to their citizens have been endangered, not when the community demanded that those who have rights also live up to their social responsibilities, but when this was not done.*[1]

Amitai Etzioni

Early Roots of Rights and Responsibilities

Even in the earliest days of recorded civilization, the relationship between healers and patients was structured and provided patients with rights. The Code of Hammurabi is the oldest known example, and it is not unlike today's quality-controlled, cost-managed and patient rights environment. It established the relationship between the healers and the patients of the day. It held physicians accountable for bad clinical outcomes. It regulated access to care. It also set compensation.[2]

It is believed to be based on even older—3000 BCE—practices. If that is true, managing the business relationship between healers and patients has been a long-standing practice in human history. American health policy didn't invent it with rules, regulations and appropriations. It seems, though, that even after 5,000 years of practice, we still can't seem to get it right. Perhaps that will bring some comfort to those in managed care today. Perhaps it will be both humbling and enlightening to those of us in health policy circles. Apparently, we have not been as creative as we believed about structuring health care. It is not as easy as we might have hoped. Our thoughtful health care management plans and proposals are nothing more than the clinical and business relationship patterns established millennia ago, and we are still working to achieve the most palatable refinements. Our health care enterprise today is much more complex, but it does not operate much differently when it comes to the fundamentals.

The Healer's Accountability for Quality

Like their older counterparts, healers today are accountable. Physicians, nurses and pharmacists have been monitored and measured from the earliest days of regulation in this country. They have taken exams, disclosed personal information and been subject to state licensing board reviews and Inspector General investigations. They have also been tracked in a National Provider Data Bank (NPDB) and monitored for malpractice experience. Hospitals and other institutions are assessed by the Joint Commission for the Accreditation of Health Care Organizations. In ancient times, governments sometimes took over the production of herbals to assure their purity. Today, the quality of pharmaceutical and medical device products are monitored by government agencies to assure the quality of the products.

These methods to measure healer performance and hold them accountable have improved over the years, and the number of organizations doing the measuring has grown as well. The National Committee for Quality Assurance (NCQA) drives quality improvement for the employers who pay for care using its Health Plan Employer Data and Information Set (HEDIS). The Foundation for Accountability (FACCT) is developing more "outcome-based" quality measures to track patients' experiences across an entire episode of care. The Agency for Health Care Research and Quality (AHRQ) is the federal government agency with the lead in quality. It has developed a comprehensive consumer satisfaction survey (known as "CAHPS") that complements HEDIS and other clinical assessment tools and enables consumers to compare the performance of health plans and providers. Peer Review Organizations (PROs) are physician-owned quality review organizations that assess quality, and each hospital and health insurance plan has its own method to track healers as well. Public and private sector purchaser coalitions measure quality to incorporate it into contracting and buying decisions. Unlike those days of old, today we don't remove a surgeon's hand when the operation is unsuccessful, but we do remove operating privileges when we judge that too many surgeries result in bad outcomes. Physicians and others lose their licenses to practice as healers. Unlike those days of old, we don't make the physician pay for the life of the slave if one dies under his care, but we do sue physicians for lost wages and damages if patients die and the healer is judged to be at fault.

The Healer's Accountability for Access and Cost

Historically, healers also played a role in assuring access. In ancient societies, care was sometimes subsidized by the ruler, or by employers (as in the case of slaves), but healers were required to cooperate to assure access by yielding to a fee schedule. This fee schedule was not only based on the nature of the healer—surgeons were paid more than physicians and pharmacists—but also on the nature of the procedure and on a sliding scale to fit the status of the patient. Yesterday's gentlemen of rank paid more for the same services than did those who were tradesmen or slaves. Tradesmen paid fees equivalent to half of what a gentleman would pay; owners of slaves paid half again as much for care of their slaves.

Similar fee arrangements are true today. Today's "gentlemen" and "persons of rank" are the insured or the wealthy who have coverage for care or who can afford to pay out-of-pocket for care. We expect them to pay more and thus absorb the costs shifted from the uninsured and the underinsured. This is so common and so embedded in our tradition of healing that we have come to expect that the poor and the uninsured will receive care and that it will be subsidized by our healers. We have come to expect that some care will be delivered at lower prices because some patients are not economically privileged. Since the earliest days of practice, and in particular, since church councils ruled that healers, at least those associated with the religious healing traditions, should not practice medicine for profit, we have come to expect that some care would naturally be uncompensated or provided at very low rates.

There is no evidence from early times that society neglected to pay for its care. Even the religious healers of the middle-ages Christian tradition were paid. They were only restricted from profiting from their healing over and above the other tributes that were paid them by the local flock in their care. How unlike health care in contemporary America, where there is resistance to paying for the cost of medical care. Furthermore, there does not appear to have been any collective effort on the part of buyers, even when the buyer was as powerful as the emperor, to leverage buying power, or to unite to purchase jointly at better rates. Not so, today. Concern for the cost of care has led governments and employers to take steps to reduce the financial liabilities associated with health care commitments.

Increasingly, powerful buyers and buying consortia are forming to get such good, low rates that the health care infrastructure is weakening. It is harder to get appointments with doctors and dentists.

Hospitals are no longer staffed adequately for the intensity of care required by patients. Institutions are strapped for cash and unable to make improvements in the data and information systems that would support more effective care. Added costs of patient care, training and research in teaching facilities are not covered adequately. Training programs for medical residents, long supported by private and public sector payers, are underfunded. Pediatrics, in particular, has been hard hit. The best and the brightest centers of academic excellence are suffering and in danger of closing. Costs that shifted from one payment center to another years ago and that were covered by wealthier and more willing payers are in jeopardy because buyers today are prudent to the point of being stingy purchasers. Costs cannot be distributed across patients and payers refusing to pay for anything other than what they, alone, receive. As a result, research, teaching and indigent care is falling by the wayside. Investor capital is drifting away from health care, envisioning a future where returns do not justify the risks of investment. Purchasers are getting the best bargain today, but scant assurance about the infrastructure for tomorrow. Healers of old had few tools for addressing disease problems, but apparently could be well paid for it. Today's healers have the tools, but greater difficulty in applying them in such adverse payment climates.

Lack of Reciprocity in the Covenant Relationship

Today's health care climate is not only adverse in its payment climate but in responsibility as well. This, too, originates in the relationships of old. The Code of Hammurabi is consistent with other *covenants of grant*. Like the Oath of Hippocrates, there are no mentions of the responsibility of patients and family members to care for themselves and each other or mention of directions to the community to do likewise in providing for healthy environments. There are no directions or requirements for healthy living. In the case of Hippocrates, because prevention, wellness, self care and love of the body were already embodied in ancient Greek lifestyle, he may have felt no reason to mention it. At any rate, the ancient codes that are the foundation of our practices today not only insulated patients from bad outcomes at the hands of physicians, they insulated patients from the bad outcomes of their own unhealthy behavior and poor lifestyle choices. The codes also ignored the responsibilities of communities. Responsibility was shifted from the patient and community to the healer. Patients and communities reaped all the benefits and bore none of the blame.

In a society in which prevention was the norm, the healer was respected and his nostrums taken as directed, this imbalance between benefits and risks might not be so problematic. In today's climate of eroded confidence in the practice of healing, this creates immense challenges. It traps today's insurance-financed, HMO-managed healers in a maddening descent into hell, defined by customer and community expectations, but not balanced by reciprocal obligations of any sort. There is plenty of evidence to detail what the public believes is wrong and how it now holds healers, and managed care in particular, responsible for the problems. Polling, focus group, marketing study, editorial, litigation and talk show data abound. Complaints—and there are plenty of them—produce the easiest insights. Americans today are quick to comment on the length of office-visit waits, the cost of prescriptions, the conditions in nursing homes and the surliness of hospital staff. We are ready with wish lists for quick fixes, cures and easy answers to tough disease problems. Oh, and another thing, we'd rather not pay for it. Someone else should—either employers or the government—and, barring that, the providers themselves should be capable of footing the bill, especially for new developments in technology. At the same time, though, we neglect good personal health practices that could reduce the cost of care. We eat too much, smoke too much, exercise too little and take risks too often. We carry guns in the streets and in our schools. Then, we want the providers of the care to cure the sickness, at little or no extra cost. Or, so it seems.

But if patients are discontented, healers are even more so. Communities are as well. Patients deal with the frustrations of today's health care episodically. The fact is most of us are healthy for the vast majority of our days. It is a minority of us who are ill at any given time, or have chronic or terminal illness that requires constant care. Healers, on the other hand, deal with it continually, so it is no surprise that healers want changes in health care as well. Many are as dissatisfied as their patients. Their work is no longer satisfying. They wonder if their clinical education has been wasted on filling out forms, attending committee meetings and dealing with bureaucratic dictates. Managed care pioneers who believed they were on the verge of finding the solutions to health care dilemmas have been excoriated in the press, blistered in Congress and bankrupted out of business. Communities are also concerned. Health care costs, unemployment, teen pregnancy, violence and guns have taken a toll on community life and drained resources from the coffers that would otherwise support education, the arts and business development. Not only are some people unhealthy, some communities are unhealthy as well. At a time when the armamentarium for clinical care and public health is at its best and positioned to add value to life and years, it isn't clear who should make the first move to create the necessary changes that will re-inspire confidence and rebuild relationships.

Limitations of the Current Covenants of Grant

We're stuck in these doldrums because our health care system today has not progressed beyond ancient times in an important way—our health care system is still a *covenant of grant* in which patients and communities receive from, but do not reciprocate with, their healers. It is a covenant of grant in which health care coverage further insulates patients and communities from the financial consequences of unhealthy behaviors. It is a covenant of grant that reinforces a dependency on healers that is frightening in its implications as the population ages. Making changes will be difficult because the covenant of grant has been further entrenched within the contracts of managed care.

Today's patients and communities are dependent on healers not only for health care services, but also, with the dawn of managed care and capitation, for the financing mechanisms to cover cost of the care. The patients of Hammurabi's era would have considered the economic costs of a clinical visit. Today's patients with third-party coverage or in managed care have few such worries. What we as patients have gained in access, we have lost in incentive for personal responsibility. A mythology has arisen in our modern culture that is dangerous for healers and patients alike. We have come to believe that it is more in the interest of managed care, or the healer/payer, to care for patients, than it is in the patients' interest to care for themselves. This mythology ignores that patients, themselves, reap benefits that merit some contribution of their own time, effort or financing. It ignores the fact that some of the best health care a patient can get is not in the healer's office, but in their own homes, workplaces and communities in the choices they themselves make between visits to healers. It is not the clinical decisions healers make that create the best value in health, but the lifestyle choices patients make and communities support day to day.

The benefits of prevention are oftentimes stated in ways that promote this mythology, holding the managed care healer/payer responsible for assuring that patients take even the most clear and simple preventive measures. One HEDIS measure assesses quality according to the number of patients who receive influenza vaccines. Why should managed care be responsible for assuring that its patients are protected from flu? How far do those responsibilities reach? With information? With patient tracking and recall systems? With free vaccine? How could any adult today not know that flu is seasonal and vaccines can prevent or ease the disease? What additional information and shot clinics should managed care provide when a multibillion dollar cough and cold products industry advertises extensively each year; and visiting nurses, Wal-Mart and neighborhood pharmacies offer easy and inexpensive access to the vaccine, at a cost equivalent to a few soft drinks? Local news broadcasts track the arrival of the offending viruses. Families suffer as parents and children alike lose work and school days to the illness. Yet, how often have patients resisted and avoided even painless, low-cost, affordable items like the influenza vaccine? How is use of flu vaccine a measure of managed care quality and not patient responsibility?

Like other preventive measures, vaccines are too often viewed as benefiting the payer more than the patient. Patients too frequently say, "The payer (government, HMO or employer) should pay for my vaccine, my check-ups, my health club, my obesity medications, because it will save them money in the long run." Legislatures too frequently agree. An entire industry has developed to make cost-effectiveness calculations, and it has flourished on the notion that health care benefits accrue to payers, and managed care in particular, of a population's health care costs. This notion can reach extremes. One state legislative proposal is aimed at requiring HMOs to cover weight loss surgery at about $15,000 per patient, with the rationale that it will save money in the future by avoiding the costs of the ancillary diseases associated with obesity such as diabetes and hypertension. Surely there are other less costly strategies for reducing obesity short of radical surgery? Is it that patients will not comply with lifestyle changes? Why should it be so much in the payers best interests that even extreme solutions and doubtful procedures are mandated? Why aren't changes in behavior and lifestyle demanded of patients? These are questions of importance for this millennium.

The dependency of patients and communities on their healers, which was established in the Oath of Hippocrates, reinforced in tradition, imbedded in the culture of medicine and facilitated by today's health financing systems, has exacerbated the health care financing problems today. This dependency has transferred too much of the responsibility in health care from the patient and the community to the healer. Healers are too often assigned responsibility for all aspects of care, cure and cost. For the capitated health care provider today—and for the managed care systems that contract with employers and governments to provide care—attempting to provide care within a paradigm that expresses patient rights but not patient responsibilities is "mission impossible." By covenant and by contract, the healer is bound to care for the patient. The patient, on the other hand, is in no way obligated to reciprocate by practicing healthy behaviors or following orders.

As a result, for example, the healers are obliged to identify hypertension, counsel patients about diet and exercise, prescribe antihypertensive medicines and subsidize at least part of the cost of the drug. They are also expected to monitor compliance, remind patients to take the medicine along the way and assess the outcome of the therapy, making changes as needed. The patient, on the other hand, needs to do nothing. The patient, living within the current covenant of grant with the healer and under financing plans with his employer (or government), does not need to show up for appointments, follow the dietary or exercise advice or take the medicines. If the patient continues to come for care, the healer will be expected to repeat all the care-giving steps. If he does not come for care, the healer will be expected to find out why and encourage him to show up. When the patient has a heart attack or stroke, the healer will be expected to provide the access and quality of care for the emergency services, intensive care, surgery and rehabilitation required to ensure survival and good quality of life afterwards. And, the healer, a managed care healer, will be expected to pay for all of this within the negotiated, preferred, capitated rate.

What is the patient's responsibility? Few oaths address the reciprocity in the relationship between healers and patients. No oath addresses how to deal with the conflict in health care today over the increasing cost of care and the responsibility of patients to help control those costs. Yet those opportunities to control costs are myriad, and the implications of not embracing these opportunities are frightening for providers of care. In today's capitated world of health care, it is the healer who bears the fiscal consequences of the failure of patients and communities to practice good health behaviors. It is also the healers who have the best insights into how to reduce those costs through responsible behavior. As such, it will fall to the healers to address this issue in the individual contacts they have with patients, in the contracts they sign with managed care or health payers and in the public policy settings within communities. There are a number of targets ripe for discussion—compliance, self care, health behaviors and public health.

In 1998, HBO aired a documentary entitled "Six Months to Live," in which the patient's heroic efforts to comply with a healer's prescription were portrayed. This documentary traced the experience of people who were facing terminal illness and seeking alternative paths to healing in addition to the traditional medical approaches of their clinicians. The story of one woman was compelling. In addition to dietary, attitudinal and other therapeutic approaches, she visited a Native American healer. His prescription for her, among other things, was that she spend a night, underground, naked and alone, with Mother Earth. Her family spent that night praying for her above ground as she, wrapped in a quilt, went down into an underground, dugout space much like a small sweat lodge. The intention of the healer was that she contemplate her mortality and eventual return to the earth. It was, no doubt, an attempt to require her to deal with the fears about her eventual death, if not from this terminal condition, then from some other in the future.

The nature of the prescription is clearly unusual in the context of today's healing practices in mainstream American medicine, and so is the response of the patient. She did it. She really did it! She spent the night, naked and alone, underground. How different from many patients in this country today, who will fail to take even one antibiotic tablet per day for ten days. Studies have shown that between 20% and 30% of patients do not fill their prescriptions, and of those who do, many take incorrect doses, take medicines at the wrong time, forget to take doses and stop medicines too soon. Logic would say that this is because the cost is too great. But surveys indicate otherwise. It is more often because they doubt the effectiveness of the medicine, fear side-effects and decide they do not need it.[3]

Self care and the practice of prevention are other ways to reduce costs. These relate to controlling the most common contributors to death and health care costs: tobacco, diet and exercise and alcohol use. These behaviors drive heart disease, cancer, accidents, chronic obstructive pulmonary disease, diabetes mellitus and chronic liver disease.[4,5] They make their marks quickly on health care costs. In as short a time as 18 months, those who engage in these high-risk behaviors will use more health care resources.[6] Frequently, these factors combine and it is difficult to sort out the individual contributions of each risky behavior to the cost of care. It is clear, however, that the costs to society are high. Patients have failed to manage their health practices to control the costs associated with these conditions. Although they suffer some of the consequences in life lost or quality of life reduced, they have not suffered financially because they have been largely insulated from the costs. Healers have failed as well. Providers have not been vocal enough about the cost implications of these lifestyle choices. Payers have paid for lifestyle-induced disease. To make matters worse, payers have further removed responsibility from patients and encouraged their dependency by creating incentives for patients to practice prevention.

Smoking-related medical expenses for the 48 million Americans who smoke, for example, hit an estimated $50 billion in 1993, or about $2.04 for every pack of cigarettes sold. These estimates are believed to be twice as high when they include workdays lost due to smoking-related illnesses. Smoking is linked to heart disease, respiratory infections, chronic bronchitis, stroke, emphysema, miscarriages, low birthweight infants and ulcers. Secondhand smoke is related to asthma and respiratory problems and deaths from lung cancer and heart disease. Smoking by women has caused the lung cancer death rate among women to rise more than 400% from 1960 to 1990, making it the number one cause of cancer deaths among women, surpassing breast cancer. Overall, more than 400,000 people die each year due to tobacco-related diseases. Sixteen percent of high school students are frequent smokers, and that number has been on the rise.[7]

Add to that the costs of sedentary lifestyles and poor nutrition. In 1999, the total health costs of treating adult obesity in the United States was $238 billion—or roughly 25% of total health care costs.[8] People who are overweight are at increased risk for heart disease, stroke, cancer, diabetes and osteoporosis. Obesity is considered the cause of more than 300,000 deaths per year. Estimates indicate that from 15% to 20% of American children and 20% to 50% of adult Americans are overweight,[9] and the matter is of such great importance that the *Journal of the American Medical Association* devoted an entire issue to obesity in October 1999.[10] Pharmaceutical companies believe that obesity drugs are possibly the world's biggest market. Analysts predict that sales of obesity drugs could exceed $26 billion in the United States alone. Treating only 25% of the patients at a cost of $3 per day would generate sales at that level.[11]

Limitations of Covenants of Grant with Communities

This same covenant of grant has been extended to communities, and with similar outcomes. Communities that fail to maintain a strong public health infrastructure and address social problems are insulated from the direct and immediate health care costs associated with those decisions. Over time they suffer from lost productivity and economic growth, but the immediate consequences are largely hidden. A Harris Poll conducted in September 1999 indicated widespread support for public health measures, such as infectious disease control, immunization, safe water, air and waste disposal and education for healthy lifestyles, particularly among the best educated and most politically influential.[12] Yet even those in favor of public health programs admitted that public health measures lacked the excitement of modern medical miracles, leaving political support for funding weak. Since it's modern miracles they expect, it's modern miracles they get; and, like patients, communities pass the bill on to "others." Too frequently, communities expect that local employers who pay for care and the managed care organizations that provide it, will continue to do so, absorbing the costs of innovations as they spill from research pipelines.

New medicines, devices and surgery compete for other financial resources; in particular, the public health programs that care for communities. If adequate public health resources are unavailable, problems will become greater in the coming years and disease outbreaks will result. Food-related diseases, for example, have become increasingly common, with 76 million illnesses, 325,000 hospitalizations and 5,000 deaths each year. The odds are one in four people will become ill from a food-borne illness each year.[13] One in 25 children remain at risk from lead poisoning in the wake of inadequately funded screening programs.[14] A number of Healthy People 2000 goals were unmet, and some measures actually got worse. West Nile Virus (WNV) Encephalitis affected the Northeast in 1999. Once the crisis of new cases subsided, regional health commissioners worried aloud about how they would pay for local mosquito control programs to prevent outbreaks in future years.[15] Rabies is once again a problem. Three thousand children were exposed to a rabid goat at a travelling fair and required treatment at $1,500 each. Rabid raccoons released by hunters at a club in West Virginia have transmitted the disease to wild and domestic animals throughout the east, causing public health officials to advise that any contact with an unknown animal on the eastern seaboard must be viewed as a potential rabies contact, and tragically, causing severe injuries to at least one baby who was attacked at his home in suburban Washington, D.C.[16] Air pollution continues to cause an estimated 50,000 to 120,000 premature deaths and $40–50 million in health costs annually from exposure to outdoor pollutants.[17] An outbreak of avian H5N1 influenza in Hong Kong recently alarmed the world medical community and demonstrated our vulnerability to a major outbreak. For influenza experts, this drove home the need to prepare for an expected pandemic. Since they are fully aware that there will not be adequate supplies of vaccine, some communities, particularly in areas of poverty, will be disproportionately adversely affected. The implications for physician and hospital costs are clear.

Besides shoring up the public health infrastructure, there are other notable social health targets. As a result of the failure to address the social issues of teenage sexuality, the U.S. has the highest teen pregnancy rate among developed countries. About one million teens become pregnant each year—95% are unintentional and one-third end in abortion. Cost of teenage pregnancy: $120 billion from 1985 to 1990. Forty-eight billion dollars could have been saved if the mother had waited until she was 20 to bear a child.[18] Other infants, more than 2,000 each year, are born with fetal alcohol syndrome (FAS), which causes growth retardation, facial abnormalities and central nervous system dysfunction. Children can suffer lifelong consequences from in utero alcohol exposure from their mother's drinking, which has risen four-fold between 1991 and 1995. In 1992, the National Institutes of Health (NIH) estimated the annual cost of FAS from mental retardation to be $1.9 billion.[19]

Despite public health programs and a new endeavor to apply epidemiology to the problems of injuries, they are not the most frequent causes of death, but they are among the most costly to the economy. Including homicide and suicide, injuries are the leading cause of years of potential life lost before age 75. The cost of injuries from automobile accidents, firearms, falls, fires, poisonings and drownings is $260 billion. Of that amount, $69 billion (in 1993 dollars) was spent on health care costs to care for injury victims. That is 12% of all medical spending.[20] Injuries account for 46% of all emergency department costs, 10% of all hospital costs and 16% of all outpatient costs.[21] Traffic crashes continue to be a leading public health problem and are still the leading cause of death for people aged 6 to 27, at $150 billion total economic costs a year.[22] Despite widespread education and the availability of free car seats, 40% of children ages 1 to 4 years are still unrestrained and nearly 80% of safety seats are improperly secured.[23] The rate of death from firearms in the United States is more than eight times that of other economically developed nations and the costs are also high. In 1990, firearm injuries cost over $20.4 billion in direct and indirect costs of health care, long-term disability and premature death. At least 80% of those costs are paid by taxpayers.[24] Finally, in 1991, the costs associated with head injury or death from head injury due to bicycle accidents was $3 billion. It is believed that 75% of bicycle-related fatalities among children could be prevented if all children wore helmets. Every helmet worn saves this country $395 in direct health care costs and other costs to society. If 85% of children wore helmets for one year, the medical savings are estimated to be between $109 million and $142 million. One person who survives a head injury may cost $4 million in health care services over a lifetime.[25]

As individuals and communities, when we fail to address these drivers of health costs, the burden is shifted to payers and healers. Payers are increasingly resistant to covering these costs and require that the healers bear the fiscal consequences of our illnesses and injuries. Too many of us prefer not to care for elderly parents, and turn to healers to do it for us. We choose to allow guns on the street, keep guns at home and at school, repeal or fail to enforce helmet and traffic laws and turn to healers to provide us with emergency care to tend our critical injuries. When we survive the accidents our risky behaviors have caused, we turn to healers at rehabilitation centers to restore lost function to damaged limbs and brains. When we fail to address the social issues driving teen pregnancy, we want healers to provide the neonatal intensive care that will keep our low birth-weight grandbabies alive—and they will. Healers are fast running out of strategies that control costs by tinkering with their own systems, however. In the future, patients and communities will need to take responsibilities for health approaches that will yield the desired cost-management results. Accepting personal responsibility, understanding risk in the population, developing targeted group interventions, case management and multidisciplinary teams that will deal with social, juvenile justice and education problems will be required. These programs will be invasive in the life of the individual and the community, but they will be necessary if we are to address the real needs of health and health care in the future.

Unfortunately, nowhere in the discussion of the modern miracles of medicine have healers confronted their individual patients, communities, or the nation as a whole with the true cost of the behaviors contributing to health care inflation. Likewise, nowhere do we systematically address the questions of conflicts the public must resolve as we confront the difficult issues of changing personal health and social behaviors. Even worse, nowhere have we systematically confronted that some of the changes—like gun control—will challenge values and liberties.

Rationale for Covenants of Obligation with Patients and Communities
Much of today's disease is preventable, yet all indications are that we cannot assume that even the most advantaged of the citizens in this nation will practice good preventive health or adhere to a healer's advice. Our rates of medication compliance are low, we gain weight and lead sedentary lives, adults shun immunizations, drive fast on highways and drive up costs that health care providers are expected to absorb. Over the decades of modern medical progress, healers have provided and patients have come to expect medical solutions to all manner of physical, emotional and social problems. Live a lifestyle that results in obesity, and healers have solutions for us. If they can't make us slim again, they can at least medicate the arthritis, diabetes and heart disease that will result. If we choose to delay childbearing, healers will help us conceive with fertility medicines and in vitro fertilization.

This perspective is frightening, as too often the patterns of disease associated with the aging population have been taken as uncontrollable givens. In fact, they are not. Patterns of disease can change as patients and communities modify behaviors and improve public health systems. Patterns of disease had better change if we are going to retain employer-based systems of financing and solvency in federal programs like Medicare. As long as the nation avoids confronting the responsibilities of patients and communities, health care today will be on the verge of a crisis that cannot be resolved with mere tinkering of per-member-per-month financing formulas, tighter Diagnosis-Related Group (DRG) payment rates, patient rights legislation, or HMO litigation.

How is this a matter of covenant? In much the same way that the divine edicts to Moses in Leviticus defined interrelationships in the life of the tribes of Israel, these questions present similar issues to us today. Our living together, sharing common water, shelter, storage and sewage enables our sharing of common plagues and bad habits. Those who choose to practice bad public health habits place the health of their neighbors at risk. Unvaccinated individuals transmit preventable diseases to others, which is a consequence for the community, not just for the unvaccinated individual. Food service workers with lax hygiene transmit Hepatitis A to their customers. Areas with contaminated ground water transmit E. coli 0157:H7 to children at state fairs. Towns without animal control operations leave their babies vulnerable to attacks by rabid raccoons. Polluted air keeps asthmatic children and adults from work and school. Drunk drivers and gun-toting teens kill others in their path.

In addition, we not only live together, we pay our health care bills together. Payers, and in particular managed care, might feel the first pinch, but ultimately, the buck stops with every worker and every taxpayer. As a result, we are jointly financially responsible for the costs of each other's healthy or unhealthy behaviors. Whether we pay taxes, buy insurance or pay for care out of our pockets, the costs of irresponsible personal and health behaviors that increase the costs of care are borne by everyone. Risk in health care financing is never "assumed," it is "spread." As a result, few patients pay the true cost of their own health insurance or their own care. Those who do pay—whether through insurance payments, lower wage rates, out-of-pocket payments or taxes—bear the costs, to some degree, for all the care that is delivered—for other taxpayers and insured persons, but disproportionately for those whose high-risk behaviors result in high-cost care. The young person, insured or not, who rides a motorcycle without a helmet and suffers an accident most likely incurs high costs in the course of his care. Even if the costs initially are borne by insurance, it is unlikely that insurance payments will be sufficient to cover them all. If, as is the case in so many high-risk/high-cost behaviors, this young person requires extensive care over some long term, he would most certainly require tax-supported Medicaid or other indigent charity patient support. Costs, when they exceed the billings, must be passed somewhere. There may be "free care" for an individual in a particular health care encounter, but there is no "free care" for an individual over a lifetime, for a community or for the nation.

Our personal and high-risk behaviors increasingly impinge on the quality of other people's lives. Likewise, our collective decision to fund or not fund community health programs increasingly impinges on us. The most stunning advances in health have been made at the community level in the past 100 years. Increasing life span and improvements in the day-to-day quality of life were supported not by medical care, but by community public health programs and personal lifestyles. Communities must create relationships that lead to reciprocity among their members to ensure health and conquer disease. This is perhaps one of the most pressing needs in health care today.

The community covenant of healing creates reciprocal relationships between healers, patients and communities. It recognizes a reality of health care today: Not only do we relate to one another as individual patients and healers, but we do so within a context created for us with communities. What we do to protect and maintain our own good health benefits not just ourselves, but others as well. Conversely, steps taken by communities to protect the health of the public at large also have an impact on each of us as individuals. That impact might be directly related to the quality of life and health we enjoy, or it may be related to the overall cost of care that we all support. We have needs and depend on others to meet them. Others have needs and depend on us. This is precisely the reciprocity of relationship of a covenant of obligation.

Some of our most contentious public policy issues are embedded in community covenants. Resolving them will require that the nature of the other covenants be acknowledged, in place and practiced. There is no other way to address the critical challenges that the advances in medical technology and patient demand place upon us. Some of these public policy issues are simmering on Main Street. Others are boiling in the halls of Congress. Still others have spilled over to Wall Street. They are the most ripe for change on matters regarding patients' rights.

The Patients' Bill of Rights

We are not facing these issues as much as we are backing into them. The health care world of the future is one in which costs will increase because of technology, demand and demographics. It is one in which patients and communities are likely to remain dependent on healers. It is one in which, along with the mythologies of health care financing, we will add the fallacy that much of the new demand for services will be absorbed into previously negotiated capitation rates. Health policy "wonks," managed care executives and some employers know we're at the breaking point. Consumers and communities, however, believe that an endless supply of health services will be available—with little demand on their wallets and even less constraint on their lifestyles.

It is into this covenant-bound and contract-driven world of health care that patient expectation, frustration and fear associated with managed care cost controls and large medical bureaucracies has finally spilled over into legislative debates. The most contentious of those are about the rights patients should have as they deal with today's healers, particularly those in managed care. Specific state and federal legislation has been debated for the past several years, proposing one sort of protection or another and as patients and, occasionally, clinicians feared, they were increasingly vulnerable to the forces of corporate medicine.

Federal patient rights debates address two principal concerns: access to care and slippage in quality, as corporate forces govern the healer-patient relationship. The list of patient rights is extensive and goes well beyond the contracts negotiated for patients by the employers and governments that arranged to pay for the care. Patients want guaranteed access to care in times of emergencies, access to specialists and access to healers from outside the plan's negotiated network. They also want access to all pharmaceuticals and clinical trials for experimental treatments. They want continuity of care when switching plans. Patients want assurances that disadvantaged groups are not discriminated against, that medical records are kept confidential, that they can get help in a confusing medical marketplace and that health plans will produce comparable information so that consumers can make better choices. They want quality. They want quality improvement processes within managed care, data collected to measure and monitor quality and utilization review programs that are rational and based on good criteria. When there are disputes about care, patients want a timely review process to settle the dispute, if necessary, by outside, disinterested parties. They want the relationship with their own physician to be protected from business intrusions. They want doctors shielded from "gag orders" that prevent candid discussions of treatments and from medical necessity guidelines that are imposed by the HMO instead of accepted by the profession. When all else fails, they want to be able to sue the administrators of the plan providing the care. These demands reached the floor of Congress because there were problems in the halls of medicine.

States have also been an active ground for clarifying patient rights, and one in which protections have not only been debated, but enacted. In early 1994 the American Medical Association developed a model law, The Patient Protection Act, that was used the following year as a guide for states' legislation. It provided the template through 1996 and was later expanded to address Managed Care Consumer Bill of Rights initiatives, which were more consumer oriented. More than half the states have adopted some type of "Patient Bill of Rights." Included in the new state laws are provisions that address continuity of care, emergency care, direct access, freedom of choice, mandated benefits, consumer grievance procedures, bans on gag clauses, bans on financial incentives, provider protections and provider profiling. Freedom of choice was a legislative proposal in 22 states, and mandated benefits were enacted in 26 states, requiring coverage of particular treatments and prescriptions. Financial incentives to compensate providers for ordering minimal care for patients are now banned in 25 states. Continuity of care legislation in 22 states addresses the problem of continuity when the individual's provider is terminated, disenrolls or if the enrollee changes HMOs. In 42 states, emergency care legislation ensures that managed care organizations provide some type of reimbursement for the cost of emergency care services. In 37 states an individual may select an OB/GYN as their primary care provider, in three states individuals are permitted to use their chiropractor as their primary care provider and in two states dermatologists can be considered as a primary care provider.

Harnessing the Voices of Patient Rights

The most articulate voices for patient rights are among the most advantaged in our society. Although these voices represent the poor, they more often represent the interests of the employed, who, unlike the growing number of Americans without health insurance, have some form of assistance to pay for most of their care. These vocal patients don't rely on charity care or government-funded programs. Unlike the poorest and unemployed Americans, they have the income to pay for those services that are not covered at all or require copayments. In today's economy they are in stable relationships with employers, and their employers are providing a noncash benefit that, for some with personal or family illnesses, will exceed the value of their salary earnings. For those who will not experience catastrophic events, the benefit brings a certain peace of mind from knowing that the protection against potentially devastating health care costs will not bankrupt family finances.

These vocal patients are precisely the people we would anticipate might be able to accept responsibility for the condition of their health. If they are healthy, we would anticipate that they would stay healthy. They would use fitness facilities, watch their diets, get flu shots and take over-the-counter remedies well and in compliance with the label. If they are not in good health, we would anticipate they might be most able to make the behavior changes required to improve it. If they need medicines, we would anticipate that they would be most capable of following the prescription regimens or guiding their own self-care with advice from the local pharmacist. If they need more services than their insurance plan subsidizes, we would anticipate that they would be willing and able to spend some of their discretionary income on care for themselves. If they feel compassion for those less fortunate, we would anticipate that they would contribute to financing for others who cannot otherwise afford it.

We would expect those who are vocal to be the leaders in their communities. They would most probably be politically active. They would be among those we call the "elites," as we poll for public opinions. They are the people we would expect to have the best knowledge and understanding of the health care financing systems that are so stressed today. They would be capable of engaging in a dialogue to retrace how these dependencies were created and how relationships can be better structured to preserve the benefits that twenty-first-century miracles can bring us.

Amidst their dissatisfaction is an opportunity to engage them, and other Americans—patients, healers and their communities—in a discussion of how to better achieve what is most desired by everyone in promoting and assuring good health and access to health care. There is an opportunity to grow past the dependencies that are so widespread in our system today and move into the interdependencies on which everyone can thrive and realize their potential. Creating covenants that address both the rights and the responsibilities of the parties involved is one way to do that.

Creating Covenants of Obligation

Patients and communities can come to recognize that good health is its own reward and a worthwhile investment. They can come to understand that they themselves benefit much more from good health than their employers, HMOs and governments ever will. They can continue to struggle for more patient rights, care and financing, but they can also recognize that with those rights must come the reciprocity of responsibility. Communities can continue to demand more miracles in medicine, but they can also recognize the value of public health systems and fund them. Communities can

---

work to improve public safety, prevent disease and not shift the burden of illness to the healers in clinical practice. The nation can continue to expect efficiency and effectiveness from its healers, but it should balance any demands with expectations that patients will accept their responsibilities as well. This will be possible, if patients, communities and the nation will reconsider covenants in health care, moving from the current *covenant of grant* and into *covenants of obligation* in healing.

These covenants of obligation would build on the existing covenants of grant and call for change in a number of areas. As in the case of any covenant, only the parties to it can adequately define its terms. Only healers, patients and their communities will be able to specify what they expect from each other and how they will agree to abide within the covenant relationships they will establish. It would be presumptuous to offer more than a directional paradigm here, but some items are clear and called for implicitly within the dissatisfactions expressed by patients, healers and communities today.

A covenant of obligation, with its rights and responsibilities, would address each of the players—the healer, the patient and the community—and their mutual, interlocking relationships. A covenant would recognize that the health of the individual is dependent on the behavior of the individual patient, the healer and the community. Likewise, the success of a healer's practice depends on the individual patient, the healer and the community. The health of the community depends on behaviors of the individual patient, the healer and the community. For example, a patient will remain healthy to the degree that he has access to quality care, takes the advice of the healer and lives in a community that provides safe water and streets. A healer's practice will yield successful results to the degree that the healer maintains a level of skill, has patients who follow medical advice and practices within a community that provides financing for patient care—whether through employers or with public funds for those who cannot otherwise afford to pay. A community's health will be assured to the degree that patients follow good health practices, healers peer-review the quality of the care rendered and the community invests in prevention and public health measures. Other aspects of these interdependent relationships will lead to the health that the patient, the healers and the community strive for, but those can only be determined if all the parties work collaboratively to make the choices about their mutual responsibilities to the others.

- Patient responsibilities. For their part, patients might asses the personal, family and social problems they face in today's society. They cannot unilaterally resolve all the problems that may contribute to their diseases and drive their need for health care resources, but each individual and family can make inroads towards improving the quality of their lives and their health. They can take personal steps to get the information they need—it is widely available today—and they can take the steps to change their behavior. They can also become politically active in creating community change of the social problems that threaten their health and safety and drive health care costs. Patients can reconsider how to balance their expectations of healers with their own responsibilities for health. Patients might thoughtfully examine whether they expect the skill of their healers to compensate for the lifestyle risks that cause disease and disability. Patients might actively seek healers who will encourage interdependence in the healing encounter.

- Healer responsibilities. For their part, healers might now draw on the vast public health literature with its information on how to prevent illness and improve health, and engage both patients and policymakers in a discussion of how to better address the patients' responsibilities. Healers might challenge why, wittingly or not, national policy has played into the current dependency dynamics, creating cost-quality access tensions that are impossible to resolve. Healers might question why patient rights bills are silent on the matter of patient responsibilities. Healers negotiating contracts with health payers might assure that the plans are written to make patients more responsible for their own lifestyles that create illness and drive medical expenditures.

- Community responsibilities. For their part, communities might reconsider the nature of the public health and social infrastructure that supports the health of individual citizens and the community at large. There is some evidence that many communities are beginning to do just that. More should. Communities might find the way to support public health programs, educate legislators and public administrators and improve funding, even in the absence of "crises." Communities might assure that public health programs are not de-funded when they are successful. Communities might resolve the social issues that drive health care costs, exploring the role of schools, families, businesses, law enforcement and the churches in working to reduce the drivers of healing costs.

- Policymaker responsibilities. For their part, policymakers and legislators might consider the dynamics of addressing issues this complex in political settings. The national and state governments that shepherd decisions on questions like these—if they are posed at all, and they rarely are—are geared to giving constituent voters the most for the least tax dollars. As a result, when the questions are posed, the answers yield not a balance among tradeoffs, but new benefits. Policymakers might search for other settings, off the "Hill" of politics that can more successfully resolve the tensions in health care today. If there are none, if politics is too intractable a venue, they might explore how politicians can avoid further entrenching the dysfunctional policies that promote today's dependencies and remove responsibility from patients and communities. Legislators might call a moratorium on mandated benefits until those mandates are coupled with patient and community responsibilities. Legislators might balance the responsibilities of managed care with rights for those organizations. They might, for example, allow managed care organizations to hold communities responsible for a portion of costs incurred for care when a public health failure results in widespread disease.

Can we bring a set of rights and responsibilities back into balance? Can we shift our expectations from one of total dependency on our healers to interdependency with them to assure the best in access, quality and cost for everyone? The answer to these questions is yes, but only if we succeed in creating something new in society's healing enterprise—a true covenant of obligation in which the relationships offer rights, but require responsibilities. This will require a level of reciprocity among patients, healers and communities. For patients this will mean a new way of living their lives and accepting responsibility for their health. For healers, it will mean shedding the parental role, and some of the power and prestige that goes with it. For communities it will mean entering into new ventures of health and healing. For everyone it will mean creating, for the first time in American health care, a truly new covenant in healing.

Chapter 4

Curing Disease

Covenant in the Animal Research Conflict

I am writing a report on animal abuse. Please send me materials about what you do.

Dear Researcher,
I admire your dedication. Your ability to help people is really amazing. I hope one day to be someone like you. You have saved many lives. Thank you.[1]

Letters from children to an association for biomedical research

Recognizing Needs and Filling Gaps

There are healers that patients rarely see. They are the researchers that explore the unknowns of the human body and push the limits of science in search of cures. Some work at the bedside, others work at the bench. Regardless of whether they ever treat patients successfully, their search for the answers to the challenges of disease makes them valuable assets in medicine today. Many of them are physicians and ascribe to a physician's oath, but even those who have not formally taken an oath operate within a covenant of sharing knowledge with their peers for the benefit of the patients they seek to help.

For all the largesse of researchers and the cures that they have provided us in modern American medicine, there are still quite a few diseases that can neither be prevented nor cured. The healers who treat us and the researchers who have developed the treatments have tremendous expertise. But even so, some of the therapies they have developed to prevent, treat or cure our ills are expensive, painful, distasteful and difficult to comply with.

Whether scientists make advances to discover new, less expensive, more palatable solutions for our suffering will depend on a number of factors. Key among them will be our support of researchers' work and innovation. We support innovation through investments in biomedical research, adequate reimbursement for new and better alternatives and a good supply of well-trained researchers working in well-equipped laboratories. After that, we rely on the hard work of those healers among us who have chosen the path of discovery, the advancement of knowledge and the serendipity of science.

We have debated and lobbied each of these various ways to support innovation since government entered the biomedical research world in mid-century. The government contributed to research in a number of ways: providing research funding to agencies, training researchers and hiring them. The government also granted rewards to the private sector for engaging in discovery. As the government gradually assumed the funding role of wealthy individuals and philanthropic foundations, the matter of biomedical research became a public domain. Research was conducted principally through the National Institutes of Health, though it was also conducted by other agencies, including the Centers for Disease Control and Prevention, and the Departments of Agriculture, Labor and Defense. Public funding allowed all eyes to focus on the nature of research in public institutions, its funding and its management. It allowed us to peer into the organizations, politics and personalities that guided research for the nation. As discovery in the private sector was recognized as important, public policy supported innovation. Through the tax code, patent laws, purchasing decisions and trade policy, rewards could be granted to those in the private sector using private capital to create the discoveries that would benefit the public. It was in the nation's interest to ensure that the research ideas and resources flowed freely into the search for cures and the improvement of health. The implications and the dollars at stake were substantial.

As a result, through its public, private and not-for profit institutions, the nation invested a small portion of its total health care spending—but still a hefty amount of funds—into its research enterprise. Total biomedical research funding in 1997 from public and private sources was estimated to be $42 billion.[2] Although it was the largest amount ever invested in this country, even the smaller amounts from prior years yielded substantial progress. The span of our lives was longer and the quality of our lives better. Infectious disease no longer claimed the lives of so many of our children; surgical techniques improved outcomes and led to the wonder of human organ transplants. Research spending to develop therapies and prevent disease created benefits for the economy.

For example, diabetes research spending of $181 million resulted in savings of $1.2 billion in annual Social Security Disability payments and returned income tax dollars to the Treasury as diabetics were more able to continue working at their jobs.[3] Kidney research spending of $9.8 million resulted in drugs that save $93 million annually in other health care costs.[4]

The examples could fill this book. Research stocked our shelves with more than 5,000 prescription medicines, 300,000 over-the-counter products and countless medical devices and surgical techniques to manage our health. Research also fuels an abundant and promising pipeline for the future. At this time, over $24 billion is being spent on 500 new medicines in development for the dozen uncured diseases in this nation that currently cost us over $600 billion annually to manage and will drive medical costs even higher as the nation ages.[5] Computer technologies will create "smart" medical devices; home- and self-care demands will create new products; and molecular medicine, minimally invasive procedures and organ replacement options will become common. Research and discovery have never been more promising or meritorious of support.

Debating Research

It might seem that research ventures, as productive as they are, would constitute one of the more placid arenas of public policy. They do not. Lobbying and debates about research programs have had their contentious moments. HIV/AIDS activists fought for increases in research support in the 1980s, convinced that "low" levels of funding were the result of the bias against the groups who had contracted the disease. In the wake of their success in obtaining funding increases, a variety of other groups countered that women's health, children's health, cardiovascular health and other disease conditions were actually more widespread and more meritorious of funding than HIV/AIDS. Debates such as these could be protracted and were always political, but they rarely became truly incendiary, except with regard to one special area: research that uses animals as subjects. Whether and when to use animals in the course of making discoveries for the benefit of humans is an issue of longstanding controversy.

Controversy in research is not new or unusual. There are disagreements in virtually every aspect of research. Some of these disagreements are about the priority of the project, the level of funding for particular areas of investigation or the qualifications of a designated researcher. Others are about the inclusion or exclusion of certain age, gender or racial groups in the studies, the acceptable degree of patient risk and the nature of patient consent. The peer-reviewed nature of research helps to surface such disagreements, and by addressing the differences of opinion of the various parties to the research, those projects actually improve.

Scientists do not shy away from controversy because it is frequently productive discourse. Disagreements are eventually re-solved, largely through compromise. For the most part, these discussions yield better results of greater utility. Over time, research methods have been refined and have become more efficient, women have been included in clinical trials, drugs have been developed for children, rare diseases have been studied, consent procedures have improved and human subjects have been better protected through external monitoring of research projects. One type of research is notable because the conflict seems intractable and relationships among those who might resolve it are deterio-rating. In the dispute concerning the use of animals in research, we seem unable to resolve our differences. We cannot even agree to disagree. Instead we have come to blows. It is only in the area of animal research that investigators must face the reality that their life's work, even when it creates a cure, will certainly create escalating, violent opposition.

Coming to Terms with Animals as Research Subjects

On April 5, 1999, an estimated $2 to $5 million worth of damage and lost research was sustained by two biomedical research facilities at the University of Minnesota.[6] Vandals damaged lab equipment, spray-painted walls, smashed computers and released over 100 animals. Some of the animals were later recovered, dead or hungry, along roadsides. Press reports noted that the Animal Liberation Front claimed responsibility, and a student animal rights group held a vigil in support of the break-in several days later.

The break-in was a violation of the Animal Enterprises Protection Act, and the U.S. Senate had just passed a bill to strengthen the penalties under the Act. Would stiffer penalties be effective? Ingrid Newkirk, co-founder of People for the Ethical Treatment of Animals (PETA), thinks not. She told the journal *Nature* that the Senate action was nothing more than a "knee-jerk piece of legislation," adding: "Nobody in any social movement has ever been deterred from breaking and entering or arson because the penalties have been elevated."[7]

Incidents and attitudes such as these are typical of those who oppose animal research and create disruptions in many parts of society today. Children in elementary and high school science classes refuse to perform the types of animal dissections that were once rites of passage for their parents. Medical company executives are targeted for bombings and are followed as they drive home at night. Researchers, their families and neighbors are attacked and harassed at home and at work. Protesters march outside government and university research facilities, sometimes breaking in, releasing animals and destroying research records. It's enough to make some researchers want to quit—and some have.

In news reports, school children and Hollywood personalities are highly visible, but it is biomedical researchers who are the most vulnerable and who bear the day-to-day consequences for our society's disagreements over animal research. They bear the burden of the nation's failure to address these disputes immediately and tangibly. Sick people suffer, too, though not always visibly and rarely immediately. Anyone today who lacks an inexpensive, palatable, readily accessible prevention, treatment or cure for which an animal model is key to the discovery or development of the therapy suffers as a result of these disputes. Even people who are healthy today are affected, as everyone can anticipate that someday they are likely to need cures that will flow from research using animals. Any employer or health care payer that funds care for unrelieved disabilities or pays for palliative care where there are no cures also suffers. Although it is not widely recognized, most people and health care payers are affected by our unresolved conflicts over the use of animals in research.

Addressing the Tensions and Conflicts

Can we engage in a reasoned and rational debate about the use of animals in the biomedical research endeavors that advance medical discoveries? Should we be willing to use animals for research, including the dogs and cats that so many of us see as near-human companions, in experiments that are painful or in ways that restrain them in laboratories? How long will we tolerate animal experimentation while we search for alternatives to animals? Will we stop research in most disease areas because the nature of some animal research is repugnant to some of us? Will patients with today's incurable diseases be allowed to have a voice in these decisions about animal research? Can we resolve this issue peacefully, or will violence continue to hound the biomedical research community? These are the questions we must address together as we move into this century.

Yet as a society, we have failed to address these tensions. As a result, those healers who have dedicated their careers to research are under fire. Skirmishes and wars surround them and there is no demilitarized zone to ensure their safety. There is no truce on the horizon, much less the promise of peace. There are neither cease-fires to anticipate, nor sanctuaries wherein to live and safely conduct research until a treaty is negotiated or animal replacements found. Worse, in the failure of our society to confront this issue, we have turned a blind eye to those who will ultimately bear the brunt of our inability to resolve this conflict: the patients.

How did this happen? Will groups opposing animal research succeed in one of their goals—to end animal research by the year 2020–2030? What will happen to patients who rely on the discoveries that animal research enables? What is the impact of demonizing those on whom scientific progress depends? What perspectives of each side in this debate would enlighten the other? What motivates animal rights groups that might enliven our covenants with each other? What does this have to do with the covenant? Are other beings on the planet—animals in this case— parties to the covenant as well? If animals have rights, do they also have obligations? Does the covenant between researcher/healers and patients supercede any other covenant that other beings might enjoy? Might perspectives on covenant be helpful in resolving these disputes?

Ethical and Moral Views Differ

To those *animal rights* advocates who oppose animal research, covenant—or some notion like it—is precisely at the heart of the issue. They believe all living beings—trees, animals, fish, birds and humans—enjoy equal rights to inhabit the world undisturbed. In the minds of *animal research* advocates, they do not.

Animal research advocates believe that because of the human being's ability to ascertain and behave in "higher" moral ways, human beings have greater authority to oversee all life. This authority extends to preserving and advancing life, even at the expense of sacrificing some lower forms of life for the good of humans. At the extremes, the lines are clearly drawn between the two camps—the animal research camp and the animal rights camp. It is easy to see that they hold different views.

The conflicts between these two camps have become deeply

rooted in ethical issues with social and cultural biases. These issues have evolved over time. They also reflect economic realities. In 1860, for example, more than 90% of all Americans lived and worked on farms, caring for and using animals to generate a livelihood. Today, that number is closer to 2%.[8] Any direct experience with the care and use of animals as sources of our food and clothing is virtually gone. In the experience of the average American today, food comes from the grocery store already butchered, cleaned, packaged and even precooked; clothes come off the rack; and animals are not tools to be used, but furry companions with near-human qualities who are to be cared for, loved and respected.

In the case of companion animals, views about their purpose and personalities are clear. We care for our companion animals very well. We purchase toys, clothing and health insurance for them. We book appointments at salons for their grooming and pleasure. We use them as surrogates for children in childless marriages and as companions in single households. Some have even become "healers" of a sort, visiting the sick and the elderly in Pet Partners programs intended to bring therapy, comfort and companionship. They have become so important to us that we grieve their deaths and seek therapy to recover from such a loss.

Adaptations to a Changing Society
Other changes have taken place over the last one hundred years as well. Animals became less important for our livelihoods but more important to our life spans. As research methods and opportunities progressed, animals advanced human life by providing biological models to explore diseases and cures. Medical science, as it developed, began to use animals in much the same way as the family farmer, who acted on the belief that God—as reflected in the Judeo-Christian tradition—gave humans dominion over animals and plants for human welfare. Using animals to benefit humankind, therefore, was seen as the true and correct order of things in life, as ordained by a higher power.

The ideology of animal research supporters is based on traditional Western values: Human beings are inherently good and have the moral authority to make decisions about natural resources; scientific advancement is positive; profit is desirable; and economic expansion is important for the continued evolution of the human race. This view does not condone needless pain and suffering, or even death, of the research animal, but it does not avoid the unpleasantness of such tasks if the benefit is to save the life of a human. These views are in direct opposition to those in the animal rights camp.

The underpinnings of the animal rights supporters are traced to a different view of the world. In this view, human beings are not the pinnacle of creation, but are one of many creatures who are part of a balanced ecological system. Further, the very characteristics that make animals, and primates in particular, ideal research subjects are the same characteristics that should protect them from research risks. Primates, ideal because they are so like humans, deserve the same protections as humans. Specifically, animal rights proponents believe that the biblical approach of human dominance over nature promotes "speciesism," that is, preferring one species to another in the natural order of things, thus bringing nature out of alignment. They counter biblical notions with claims that Jesus was a vegetarian and would have granted animals their rights. Ingrid Newkirk, the most often quoted authority on animal rights views, has said: "Animal liberationists do not separate out the human animal, so there is no rational basis for saying that a human being has special rights. A rat is a pig is a dog is a boy. They're all mammals."[9]

It is not only in the area of research on animals, however, in which we have witnessed a change in attitude concerning research subjects. Over the past century, our views of research subjects have evolved into ethics in biomedical research. In the early days of this nation, for example, national racial attitudes shaped medical researchers' views concerning the tolerance of pain. This affected research on Indians and slaves. The European races were viewed as more "hypersensitive" and, therefore, poor research subjects in studies involving pain, while Native Americans and slaves were viewed as not perceiving pain until they became civilized. As a result, a famous gynecologic surgeon in the early 1800s performed experimental operations on slave women because "Negresses . . . will bear cutting with nearly, if not quite, as much impunity as dogs and rabbits."[10] His view was common among those in the dominant culture of the day. Prior to our relatively recent ethical considerations of pediatric research, children, as well, were used as research subjects without the consent of their parents, exposing them to painful procedures, questionable experiments and fatal diseases. Nazis performed human experiments without regard to the pain or dignity of their subjects—a fact that is positioned against animal research by artist Judy Chicago in *Why Can't We Learn from the Past? Dachau/Silver Spring Study for Four Questions.* In this work, which is part of the artist's major project on the Holocaust, the high-altitude human experiments at Dachau are juxtaposed against experiments on primates at a Silver Spring, Maryland lab. Chicago states: "I keep asking: Where should the line be drawn between human experiments (which are generally unacceptable to most people) with animal experiments (which usually inflict intense suffering on the subjects but which most people accept, particularly if they 'save human lives')."[11]

Sophisticated Strategies Emerge

The animal rights groups promote their ideology in a variety of ways, and quite effectively so. Since animal rights groups tend to be more heterogeneous than the animal research groups, they can draw upon a wider variety of tactics for meeting their goals. This enhances the probability of their success. Some are peaceful, others are not. Those that are the most extreme tend to share belief systems anchored in socialist, equality-based views of the world. The more violent have links to the environmental movement and to terrorist organizations—something that is well documented internationally and followed by the Federal Bureau of Investigation. They share some traits with radical groups, as demonstrated by the statements of the most extreme of these activists. These groups view the use of animals akin to the abuse of humans. They see it as so entrenched that only a radical transformation of existing power structures and human consciousness can bring an end to it.[12] For these individuals, animal rights is a cause within a cause. Until the roots of the abuse are weeded from society, there can be no compromise.

Because the groups are so varied, some can act under cover of the others. Those that are violent can work with those that are peaceful to push the limits of their common agenda. The general public, for example, believes that the Humane Society is a small, local operation of volunteers who shelter and neuter stray animals. In reality, however, the Humane Society of the United States (HSUS) is a powerful, politically active, national organization that is not affiliated with any local animal shelters or humane organizations. The HSUS operates nine regional offices and is the nation's largest animal protection organization, with more than 5 million members. HSUS promotes humane stewardship in the use of animals in factory farms, fashion runways, circus tents, rodeo shows and local animal shelters.[13] But it also spends millions of dollars lobbying to eradicate a major segment of biomedical research that is dependent on animals. Although its activities are not violent, its leadership has grown more radical over the years, and some of the more extreme activists align themselves with HSUS initiatives.

Securing Public Support

Animal rights groups have positioned themselves as caring individuals who are knowledgeable about the irresponsible practices of researchers. They also claim, and have been able to sustain due to the absence of compelling counter-claims, that there are alternatives to the use of animals in research. The decision of a consumer products company as significant as Proctor and Gamble to eliminate animal testing confirms this view.

Animal rights groups have mastered the sound bites of modern communications. Further, and most interesting, they have a favorable public image. Despite the presence of terrorists within their ranks they are perceived as reasonable, compassionate individuals. Terrorist actions, such as threats against researchers and research lab break-ins, occur with relative frequency. Hundreds have been recorded over the last ten years, and in the last year alone militant activists have destroyed years of research and caused millions of dollars in damage to facilities. Yet animal rights groups have not lost favor with the public. They are very effective in securing public sympathy.

Animal rights groups are also effective in securing public policy support. They use litigation to increase lawsuits against animal research facilities. They use regulation to increase inspection of research facilities and reduce the use of certain species in biomedical research. They use state, local citizen and parent participation in educational curricula to eliminate animals in science dissection lessons. They raise the barriers for the use of animals in public and private research centers, requiring ever greater care of those animals. They make communications about animal research increasingly difficult and risky. Though some tactics, taken individually, may seem trivial, collectively these incidents amass momentum and visibility and create precedents for new animal research barriers. Here are some examples:

- On April 21, 1999 the Supreme Court denied a petition appealing a federal appeals court ruling that gave human beings the right to sue on behalf of animals. This gives animals a standing in the judicial system.

- The Animal Legal Defense Fund ties up researchers' time

and funds by suing the research community. Their intention is to do this so often that researchers "won't know what courtroom they are supposed to appear in that day."[14]

- The Great Ape Project, backed by the Animal Legal Defense Fund, was a ballot initiative to give Great Apes human rights in New Zealand. Because New Zealand has no Great Apes, it was chosen as the location to initiate this change in public policy on the assumption that no interest or opposition would surface from the public. The initiative has failed so far, but if it succeeds it will create the first policy of its type and will set a precedent for similar policy efforts in nations that do have Great Apes.

- In the United States, the 1966 Animal Welfare Act applies to all research facilities that use animals designated by the U.S. Secretary of Agriculture, including guinea pigs, hamsters, gerbils, rabbits, dogs, cats, nonhuman primates, marine mammals, farm animal species when used in biomedical research and warm-blooded wild animals. Laboratory rats, mice (except field mice) and birds are not covered. The HSUS has petitioned the U.S. Department of Agriculture to add laboratory rats, mice and birds to the list of designated animals. This would lead to annual inspections and detailed reports to account for each animal used in research. Since mice and rats comprise 90% of the animals used today, this expansion would create a substantial administrative and financial challenge for researchers.

- Finally, chimps bred in the early years of HIV/AIDS research are being phased out. Since they live up to 35 years past their time as research subjects and it is illegal to euthanize these animals, retirement communities or sanctuaries for chimps have been proposed. A task force of six animal rights groups has proposed The National Chimpanzee Research Retirement Act to advance this cause.

As radical as some animal rights groups actions might be, do they have a perspective that merits attention by the animal research culture? What steps should animal researchers take to resolve these seemingly intractable conflicts? Will the views of animal rights activists today represent yet another step in the evolution of human compassion? The attitudes and experiments performed on humans in the past one hundred years would be unimaginable today. Will we look back one hundred years from now and view this era as horrific for its use of animals? Is there a way to capitalize on the compassion, dignity and humanity expressed in the animal rights views? Should there be greater protections for animals? Can we move more deliberately to create alternatives to the use of animals in research? Can we protect animal research in the meantime? Can we find alternatives, not just for the benefit of the animals, but for the researchers and patients as well?

Defending Animal Research

Animal research defenders have so far proven to be no match for their opponents. The efforts of the opposition are successful and increasingly easier because the political landscape of the nation has shifted on this issue. The political environment has become more favorable toward the animal rights ideology as mainstream America has moved center-left on issues such as this. It is no longer easy to counterbalance the varied tactics of the animal rights groups within such a receptive environment. As a result, biomedical researchers, particularly those supported by for-profit health care companies, cannot be as vocal in defending animal research as they once were. The changed landscape makes their politically incorrect views risky, especially in the context of today's disengaged public. The good intentions of researchers and even the clear, unmet needs of patients are not persuasive.

Animal research groups face other challenges also, and as a result are no match for the tactics of their animal rights opponents. Communication plans are underfunded and are too diffuse to counter the specific targets of the animal rights groups. Animal research groups tend to be smaller, more homogeneous in their make-up and more similar in their tactics. They tend to focus on education and information about the value of research, science and discovery. In the course of their educational messages, they provide information about those projects that use animals, but animal research is by no means their only message, thus the animal use components of the message are diluted. Academic, government and private-sector researchers are active in these educational and legislative lobbying projects in partnership with groups such as the National Association for Biomedical Research (NABR). They join state-based groups similar to NABR to educate school children and teachers on the importance of scientific discoveries in an effort to balance the antianimal research messages now actively promoted to children by the animal rights groups. These activities are intended to help maintain whatever opportunity the animal research community has left, as the animal rights ideology progressively gains ground, but unfortunately, they distract researchers from a life's mission to discover cures and place researchers at even greater risks of retaliation.

Even these limited educational activities are vulnerable, however. Animal researchers are caring, compassionate, committed and hardworking. Some are eloquent and passionate spokespeople. But most are afraid to speak out on the issue. Frankly, passion and commitment alone will not stem the tide of increasing barriers to animal research. The animal research community has attempted to identify and promote alternatives to the use of animals in research. Johns Hopkins Medical School houses the principal center for the study of alternatives, and numerous other groups in the private sector are seeking, albeit in limited ways, to end their use of animals. The National Institutes of Health and a number of health care companies have provided funds for such purposes.[15] Alternatives are emerging, and some are adequate replacements. There are not yet enough animal alternatives for use in the lab, however; or are those alternatives adequate to demonstrate safety and efficacy to the Food and Drug Administration (FDA) in compliance with its regulations for drug or device development and approval. Until the alternatives are accepted by the FDA, animal research must continue. Frankly, even the tangible products of their efforts—the medical discoveries, surgical procedures, pharmaceutical products and insights into behavioral and physical mysteries—may not be enough. The balance between the rights of animals and the needs of patients has not been met, and the dynamics are tipping the scales away from research.

Engaging the Covenant

Unless a more productive dialogue is engaged between the animal rights and animal research communities, and unless patients and other healers become parties to the discussion, the animal rights effort is steaming ahead toward success in ending research on animals. The politics, the ethics, the economics and the harassment will likely drive researchers and the use of animals out of the research enterprise.

The result of such an outcome is not yet fully clear. Even today, animal research groups would like to reduce and, to the degree possible, eliminate the use of animals in their studies. Their long-term goals are similar to those of the animal rights groups. Animals are an expensive way to gain new knowledge and researchers are not, at heart, sadistic. It is the short-term goals of the researchers that are at odds with those of the animal rights groups.

Researchers are not able to eliminate animals from studies at this time because there are not sufficient, legitimate alternatives. Regulatory agencies that approve products used by humans, and even by animals in their clinical care, do not sanction nonanimal models as proof of safety and efficacy.

Given that both animal rights and animal research interests agree on the long-term objective, it seems that the issue is not one of *whether* science will end research on animals, but *when* and *how*. The HSUS initiative to end research involving unrelieved pain and distress in animals may or may not be met by its 2020 target, but the likelihood of ending all animal research at some future time is certain. It is likely that our children, or theirs, will live in a world in which researchers will not be using animals to explore health and disease. Alternatives will be sufficient and regulatory requirements will be adjusted accordingly.

How will we continue discovery in the meantime? Will scientists continue to work under fire or will we come to peace? Who will tell today's impatient patients that they will not have treatments and cures for what ails them because the quality of an animal's life is more important than their own? How will we explain to our children that their diseases of middle and old age may not be treated for lack of knowledge and products? Conversely, how can we tell them that we allowed the research procedures that so many of them considered barbaric? How will new drugs be developed and proven safe for testing in humans if they have not yet been tested in animals? Can we accelerate the search for alternatives to animals? Will the nation provide better protection for its researchers/healers who use animals until alternatives are available? If animals have rights within the covenant, do they have responsibilities? If they join in the covenant, who will speak for them in creating and sustaining their reciprocal responsibilities to humankind? How do we engage the balance and seek the proper course within the covenant of care and discovery?

We in this nation have a covenant responsibility to those patients who are ill and with those researchers/healers who seek the cures to treat them. We also have a responsibility to the large segment of our fellow citizens who feel so strongly about this issue. As a nation, we have a responsibility to hear both voices—the one that calls for caring through discovery and the one that calls for caring by ending research on animals. We have a responsibility to seek a peaceful resolution to the conflict. It would be a breakdown of the covenant of healing to allow these conflicts to threaten researchers and delay discoveries to cure disease. National leaders in research, clinical care and government should create the forums, act as the arbitrators, engage the referees and participate in the resolution. It should call upon those who are now activists to change their tactics, shift their focus, cease their violence and seek peaceful solutions.

- It is with informed debates, rather than inflammatory rhetoric and terrorist activity, that this conflict should be resolved. In the meantime, in order to facilitate a resolution, it is time for a truce on all sides and a temporary cease-fire so that a real dialogue can begin. This dialogue must address how best to continue progress in discovery while we explore alternatives to animal research.

- Each side should acknowledge the concerns and views of the other, especially with regard to commonly held views. In this debate, each side has assumed polarizing positions and has hardened those positions over time. Demonizing the other side is not a productive road to resolution at a time when reason must prevail. The reality is that the goals of the "other" are not dissimilar and their common ground is big enough for both. Both animal research and animal rights advocates would like to end the practice of conducting animal research. Joint recognition of that fact should expedite an agreement for mutual goals to identify alternatives and to institutionalize them within the research and regulatory frameworks of discovery.

- Particularly with regard to the views of animal rights advocates, it is time animal research supporters listen carefully to the messages about humanity that are embedded in the ethics of animal protection. Here, in the new millennium, those views challenge the notions of who we are as a human species and may teach us important lessons about the value of life for the next one thousand years. Those views may lead to major social changes in the allocation of resources that support children, the underserved and the elderly in ways that we do not address comprehensively in this nation or on the globe today.

- Once the opposing sides have recognized their common ground and reached an agreement on the nature of the objectives, they should develop practical steps and a joint agenda for accomplishing the end goal. Doing so might include creating a timetable, a process and increased funding for such activities to reduce any unnecessary use of research animals; developing alternatives to animals;

ensuring the safety of researchers, their families, and their projects; and providing the most compassionate care of animals used in research.

- The groups should encourage responsible, mutually satisfying behavior among their members and should agree to monitor and police their own factions.

- Local, state and federal governments should assist with laws, regulation and enforcement actions that prevent and prosecute violence against researchers and property.

- Improper handling of research animals and known violations of lab animal standards by researchers should be prevented and prosecuted as well.

Years of hostility and opposition are not fertile ground on which to seek a truce, a compromise and eventual peace. It will be difficult for the opposing sides in this controversy to work together, but it is the responsibility of both sides to do so. It will be difficult to call upon those activists who have been demonized and invite them into a covenant of caring for people through discovery. I believe that it is the community of healers who must make the first move, however, and do precisely that.

In fact, there is little other choice. When healers choose to embrace covenants, they must take all necessary steps to meet their obligations within the covenant. In this case, fulfilling those obligations entails engaging opponents who disagree with views about animal research. If healers today fail to take these steps, they will have failed within the most important covenant of all: The one that heals the patients that healers are sworn to help.

Chapter 5

Making Choices

Covenant in the Tradeoffs between Privacy and Efficiency

*Just like our free speech rights, privacy rights can never be
absolute. We must balance our protections of privacy with
our public responsibility to support national priorities—like
public health, research, quality care, and our fight against
health care fraud and abuse.*

Donna E. Shalala, Secretary of Health and Human Services,
National Press Club, Washington, D.C., July 31,1997

Are patients today willing to make sacrifices to reduce the cost
of care? What kind of sacrifices would they be willing to
make? Would they forego easy access to care? Would they do
without convenient care? Comfort? Quality? Would they agree to
sacrifice some loss of privacy or confidentiality in return for better
quality at reduced costs? Would they be willing to share their
health care data so that more research could be done on the
problems of health care systems and disease? Would they be
willing to have healers phone them to monitor their personal health
practices and encourage healthier behaviors? Would they agree
to be contacted by pharmacists, case managers or medication
compliance companies when they fail to renew their prescriptions?

Tradeoffs: Privacy and Confidentiality
vs. Efficiency and Effectiveness

Questions about tradeoffs are rarely posed to the American public. Health care policymakers more often attempt to satisfy all of the
needs of patients without asking them to choose from among
desirable goals or limit wish lists. Health systems, for example,
have attempted to provide high levels of access and quality at low
cost, without sacrificing one for the others. When providers have
been unable to satisfy all of the patients' demands, the result has
been fairly consistent—anger and calls for patient rights and
protections from the seemingly capricious actions of healers. This

is the experience of managed care today, as it attempts to meet payers' demands to further reduce costs without sacrificing quality.

Without posing the question explicitly, the tough tradeoffs related to privacy and confidentiality vs. efficiency and effectiveness are now underway. On behalf of the consuming public, legislation and pending regulation are making decisions about what information will be shared, how it will be managed and whether patients will have the right to object and protect their health care information from disclosure. These decisions are being made in order to enhance the efficiencies and effectiveness of health care practices. Implied here is that patients will lose some acceptable level of privacy and confidentiality in return for some eventual financial benefits from better managed health care systems. It is one of the most difficult tradeoffs that health care will face in the new millennium, and it is being done without a clear understanding on the part of patients—or their healers for that matter—of the implications and issues involved. Congress has made some attempts to deal with it, and the Clinton Administration has advanced regulatory proposals to do so. The Congress and the Administration are unlikely to satisfy patients. Whether policy-makers opt for more privacy and confidentiality or for more efficiency and effectiveness, neither choice is likely to succeed in satisfying patients. The tradeoff involved is too deeply embedded in the Constitution and too close to our concerns for the cost of care. The choice may require that we go beyond the values we have come to hold dear as a nation. This debate will produce agonizing choices and fearful solutions. Given its current course, this debate will also produce considerable consumer backlash as patients become more acquainted with how their data is collected and used throughout the health care enterprise without their knowledge and consent.

Health care providers today are searching for every possible way to reduce costs. As healing has evolved from a cottage industry of independent physicians and hospitals to major systems of clinical care, new ways to assess care and reduce costs have appeared. Data systems that track visits and bill payers are one of those ways that can be used to better understand the nature of the patients being served. Even in an era before electronic medical records, computerized billing data was a readily available source of information about the diagnosis, the patient's characteristics and the services used to treat the condition.

Using Data to Create Efficiency and Effectiveness

Bills contain identifying information about patients: their names, addresses, telephone numbers at home and at work, Social Security numbers, insurance plan data, vital clinical history and physical information, diagnosis codes, diagnostic tests, interventions and prognosis. The treating physician is also identified, making the source and location of the medical record clear for any follow-up inquiries about that provider that might have been needed. This data is valuable for both the public and private sectors working to improve health care efficiency and data utility.

Government and employers were the first to need and use this data in order to manage their own costs and understand the needs of their own beneficiary populations. They structured uniform bills and standards for collecting the information so that it could be collected reliably and analyzed across physician practices, hospitals and regions of the country. Next, investors became important stakeholders. As those who provided capital for business growth, investors needed to determine the performance of the firms using their resources. Investors needed to assess their risks and likely returns and keep scorecards on corporate performance. As utilization and prices changed and costs grew, so, too, did the need to understand the process of delivering health care and the ways to control and improve it.

The interests in efficiency never waned, and the importance of effectiveness emerged. There were heavy demands on data. It was through data, after all, that we expected our understanding of health systems to emerge. As an ancient healer might have explored the entrails of some animal for diagnostic clues, we searched the bowels of data, looking for information that would help to manage the increasingly uncontrollable nature of health costs. Health services research emerged as a new discipline of study. New investigative methods and data handling and warehousing systems emerged to provide the tools to assess care. Patients, physicians, hospitals and regions of the nation were studied. An era of monitoring resources consumed against characteristics of the population and their diseases began. We looked for variations everywhere, not being sure what they meant, but hopeful that if we studied variations in practice patterns and utilization, the data would give up its secrets and inform us about the proper way to practice medicine. A federal agency was funded to conduct intramural and extramural research in the area of health services research and quality. It grew and became a significant player in understanding the nature of health delivery and quality in the nation.[1]

The billing data was useful in a number of ways. Physician practice patterns were identified and monitored by third-party payers. Norms for physician practices were published and used to change clinical care. Slowly, but steadily over a number of decades, guidelines emerged from the data and were disseminated. At first, these guidelines were excoriated by the profession. Later, they were accepted and even expected. New patient intervention programs also emerged using billing form data. Claims could be analyzed to determine which patients were not refilling medications so that they could be called and counseled to do so. Children who needed vaccines could be referred back to the doctor's office for shots at the appropriate times. Missed opportunities for mammograms and pap smears could be corrected. Physicians with low rates of preventive care could be educated to do better. Epidemiologists investigated patterns of disease and public health officials launched programs to prevent disease and disability. Quality committees studied hospitals and doctors to improve practice patterns. Medical science advanced, saving lives and dollars.

Patient medical records became useful for research and patient health care programs. This information was usually de-identified, so that the researchers would not know the identity of the patient. But not always. At times some users of health care data needed patient identifying information and even when identities were "scrubbed," there was a chance that reverse engineering and merging of databases could identify a patient and cause them harm from lost privacy.

Certainly, patients knew that their bills and records were being "shared" with others in health care outside their physician's office or hospital room. A statement giving physicians permission to release medical information to secure payment was printed on each reimbursement form. Similar statements accompanied applications for health and life insurance. It is highly unlikely, however, that those patients and even many physicians understood the extent to which the data would be used for other purposes. It is also highly unlikely that they knew how data warehouses—similar to the bureaus for financial data—were developing and now reselling that information to researchers. And it is unlikely those patients realized that companies were using the data to conduct health economic studies and to develop new products and services such as patient marketing, compliance and reminder programs.

As a result, it is likely that issues of privacy and confidentiality will be the sleeper controversy of the future for health care. The protections of privacy and confidentiality are taken for granted in the one-to-one healing encounter. Unfortunately, they are eroding in private practices and even more so in the corporate practice of medicine. As demands are made by patients and payers to control costs, the sale and use of health information becomes one strategy to deliver on the promise to do so. Health care businesses are taking risks with confidential data—sometimes on their own initiative and sometimes under contractual agreements with employers and payers. As they do, they are at risk because they are acting ahead of the public's concurrence. Health executives believe they have the implicit, and sometimes the explicit, authorizations to share data, but they do not. They do not because the public does not know the full extent of these practices, and it has hardly been asked whether it is willing to sacrifice privacy and confidentiality in return for (eventual) lower costs and more effective care. The public does suspect, however, that some mischief is afoot. In a recent California Healthcare Association poll of 1,000 consumers, 60% trusted their personal physicians to keep information confidential, but only 35% trusted health plans.[2] When the public finds out the full extent of the use of information, including how information is sold and used, even by those they have trusted most, they are likely to be angry. They haven't been invited to engage in a discussion of these issues or decide on this tradeoff. No issue in health care is more vulnerable to a widespread violation of the covenant today, and no issue is so vulnerable to consumer backlash as a result.

But back to the opening questions. Health care managers know that if they use the data from many individual healing encounters they can do research, improve quality and manage costs. Isn't that what patients want? Since patients rarely pay the full cost for their care, why not require that their encounter data be used as a quid pro quo for reimbursement? Over time, this would benefit individuals as well as the group. New knowledge would lead to new insights into care and cures. New methods of monitoring physician practices would lead to better fraud investigations. Costs would decline. Health care would become more efficient and more effective. Isn't that what patients and healers alike want? Perhaps not, as recent history has shown.

Privacy Goes Public
Recent public awareness of these issues flared after a front-page

article appeared in the *Washington Post* on Sunday, February 15, 1998.[3] The story was a report—and an erroneous one at that—suggesting that CVS and Giant pharmacies had sold customer—that is, patient—lists to GlaxoWellcome, a pharmaceutical company. The story reported that drug companies were using those lists to persuade pharmacy customers to buy the company's drugs instead of the drugs prescribed by their physicians. It also reported that another company, Elensys, that sends compliance and educational literature on behalf of the pharmacies, had participated in a scheme that violated the privacy rights of the patients whose records were in the pharmacy computers. The *Post* articles reported that Elensys operated marketing and "switching" programs for pharmaceutical companies, and it reinforced that accusation in a February 18 editorial. Three days later the *Post* printed a retraction buried on page 18, explaining that GlaxoWellcome did not receive patient information. The damage, however, had already been done.

The *Post* story hit the pharmaceutical industry hard and should have reverberated throughout all of health care. It was not just a single blip on the radar screen, appearing and disappearing without notice. Rather, the story was one of several important events that drove home the challenges of privacy policy and practices. Privacy concerns are real because privacy violations are real. The medical and mental health records of a congresswoman from New York were faxed to a local newspaper during her campaign. A Massachusetts HMO kept extensive notes of psychotherapy sessions on a central computer accessible to all clinical employees. Sales representatives of a managed care company in Maryland illegally purchased the computer records of Medicaid recipients from Medicaid clerks. That same database was accessed by a banker checking on the prognosis of loan customers with cancer. A medical student in Colorado sold hospital records to malpractice attorneys. In Florida, the names of over 4,000 HIV-positive individuals were obtained and sent to Florida newspapers. A purchaser of a second-hand computer discovered that the hard drive contained a grocery store's pharmacy records, including patient names, addresses, Social Security numbers and prescription medicines. In a move that privacy advocates regard as "scary," Iceland's Parliament voted in December 1998 to draw blood from each of its 270,000 residents for detailed genetic research and sell that information to Roche Holding AG for $200 million. It also gave Roche the contents of its citizens' uniquely rich medical and genealogical records as part of the deal.

It took patient advocates in Iceland a few months to respond with their objections; Americans responded in a matter of days. Patients flooded CVS with complaints, causing CVS to terminate its patient education program and Giant to halt one that it had planned. Newspapers and television stations around the country reported on the *Washington Post* story, touching off a wave of negative media publicity. Within days, a CVS customer filed a class-action suit in Massachusetts Superior Court, naming CVS, Elensys and GlaxoWellcome as defendants. That lawsuit has since spilled over to include other companies.[4] It did not matter that the media slant on this issue was not only misinformed, it was unbalanced. It did not look at the value of the educational programs or the necessity of working with patients to ensure that they took medications properly, all of which are intended to bring down the personal and societal costs of care and to improve the quality of the patients' lives. What the event did, though, was to demonstrate the volatility of privacy matters in health care. Policymakers and health cost-cutting program designers would be well advised to take note, especially as they pursue internet and e-commerce ventures that will most certainly escalate privacy awareness.

These and similar events are beginning to create the political will to deal with the tough issues in protecting privacy, though success remains elusive. The Health Insurance Portability and Accountability Act of 1996 (HIPAA) required that Congress pass privacy legislation by August 1999. Although there were five major bills in the 105th Congress, none of them passed, and Congress missed its self-imposed deadline to act. The Secretary of the Department of Health and Human Services has now issued draft regulations, despite requests from some members of Congress to delay action until they can reconsider the issues. The Administration is moving ahead on this potentially contentious issue in the absence of a solid national understanding. Long before the closing date for comments on the medical privacy regulations of the Department, it received over 40,000 comments, many of which posed unresolvable policy and operational dilemmas. It risks falling into the hands of an angry public. With more than 250 initiatives in state legislatures across the country to address patient privacy, national policymakers and health care businesses alike face a complex patchwork of patient protections that, alone, would cripple the very efficiencies that data collection seeks to achieve.[5]

Involving Patients in the Tradeoff

Would patients care? Would they be willing to allow data on their health care encounters with physicians, hospitals, home health agencies and others to be used to study health care to reduce its costs? Would they want to restrict the use of the data to researchers? Would it be acceptable if entrepreneurs used the data to satisfy a health care market interest in lower-cost care? Would they trust those who collect, house and use the data to secure it, protect their privacy and confidentiality and use it only for healing purposes? Would they want a copy of the data? Would they want to correct errors in the records? Would they want to be paid for the data if others used it for some commercial purpose?

Frankly, we don't know the answers to these questions. The American public hasn't been asked. Someone had better ask them. Patient privacy and confidentiality is one of the most difficult sacrifices patients may be required to make as health care enters the new millennium. The notion that we might lose it—and worse, that we already have—is shocking. Privacy and confidentiality, after all, was present at the birth of organized medicine. It was a tenet of the Hippocratic Oath, which states: "All that may come to my knowledge in the exercise of my profession or outside of my profession or in daily commerce with men, which ought not spread abroad, I will keep secret and will never reveal."[6] Few issues in medicine are more fundamental to the dignity of the patient and the trust required between patient and healer.

The consideration of privacy and confidentiality has so far been the turf of an elite group of attorneys and advocates who are protecting the patient's privacy rights against the corporate practice of medicine. These advocates are doing a good job, to be sure, as are those wishing to use the data, but all of them together are only a small portion of the total players who should be engaged in the discussions. Few patients themselves have been involved, and few understand the implications for their jobs, their insurance and their future. The likely outcome will be a loss of privacy and confidentiality rights for patients in favor of reducing the costs of care. As data-driven programs unfold and the devil in the details becomes more widely known, there will be hell to pay.

Some opponents of tough privacy legislation and regulation will argue that the issues are complex and that the public will not have the attention span required of participants in the debate. They may be right. Many public debates that engage the community are complex. This one will be even more so. That places an even greater burden on those shaping this policy to take the time and the care to do it right. A good place to begin on this issue is with the definition of the terms. The definitions are critical, and the terms are muddled. The definitions are especially important because the terms in this debate cannot be used interchangeably, though they frequently are.

Clarifying the Terms
Privacy is the right of the patient to have personal information kept secret and from others, including the health care providers involved in their care. Confidentiality is the protection of that information once it is disclosed from dispersal to persons not directly involved in providing care, both within and outside health care settings. Security encompasses the policy, procedures and technologies intended to guarantee privacy and confidentiality.

Suppose that a patient seeks a diagnosis for an illness and gives permission for blood to be drawn and tested for a suspected condition like high cholesterol. The patient's right to privacy dictates that the healer test only for cholesterol level and not for other conditions, such as HIV infection, drug use or genetic diseases, on its own or at the request of another party such as law enforcement, employers or insurers. Confidentiality protections would ensure that the results of the cholesterol test, once known, are not disclosed outside the patient-healer relationship without the patient's permission. Security protections would dictate how the records of the test results would be stored and managed to ensure that they do not fall into unauthorized hands.

These are not esoteric definitional distinctions. Although these issues were once the territory of academics and scholars of constitutional law, average citizens now have a stake in them. The resolution of this debate in the public arena will affect the quality of life into the next millennium. Some patients already suffer from the loss of privacy, confidentiality and security. Some patients fear, and rightly so, that mental health records, HIV/AIDS status, genetic predisposition to health conditions and disabilities may deny them jobs, health and life insurance and even home mortgages. Some fear law enforcement surveillance of medical data in cases of drug abuse, spouse abuse and child support enforcement, and these fears are realistic as information becomes more widely accessible and electronically enhanced. It is no wonder that a 1993 Harris-Equifax poll estimated that approximately 10% of health care is "off the books" to protect disclosure of medical information outside the healing setting.[7] These fears will no doubt escalate when the public, finally attending to the issues, understands that the Clinton Administration , and likely administrations to follow, proposes that anyone receiving health care insurance reimbursement should allow their records to be used for purposes other than their own personal health care.

Framing the Covenant to Address the Tradeoff

Unless the tradeoffs between health care effectiveness and efficiency and personal privacy and confidentiality are addressed thoughtfully, both patients and healers will pay the price. Patients will suffer for the probable lack of privacy and confidentiality in their care. They will feel violated if confidential information is disclosed to others and that disclosure affects other aspects of their lives. If they cannot get jobs, insurance or mortgages, the consequences for them will be real. If they avoid care because they fear the implications for their lives, the consequences will be equally negative. Healers will suffer from the disruptions to their businesses. The costs of running a health care enterprise are likely to increase as privacy protections create new demands on medical records systems and procedures, and as patients sue for real or imagined losses of privacy. Negative press will tarnish the public image of healers, particularly those in corporate healing enterprises like managed care and pharmaceuticals. That negative press will further erode the trust in the clinical relationship between patients and their healers that is necessary for good clinical care. Legislation in this arena is critical, but to date it has been buttressed by incomplete and poor policy debates that are founded on too little data on the part of both patients and their healers. All of this is likely to impair the ability of the health care system to function optimally as it attempts to address the tradeoffs involved.

Department of Health and Human Services Secretary Donna Shalala developed a set of principles that will serve as the foundation for the impending debates on privacy. Those principles dictate that health data should be protected and used only for health purposes, patients should have control over their data, patients should be willing to share de-identified confidential information for improved understanding and care management, and providers who wrongly disclose data should be punished. These principles are a good starting point, and there is widespread agreement about them. But real questions remain. How long will this agreement hold up when the debate turns to writing regulations and requiring disclosure? Few in health care today are prepared to address the devil in the details of privacy and confidentiality. Nor are we prepared to address the devil in the dollars. Implementing the confidentiality and security provisions recommended by the Secretary will at least equal the cost of Y2K compliance. With physician practices, hospitals and managed care companies operating at low profit margins, there is not much capital available to institute the variety of changes that will be required.

Regardless of the cost, the completeness and the soundness of the data sets will likely be questionable. For example, patients, in one instance in which they were asked, did not respond favorably to the sharing of their medical information. Mayo Clinic, a major, credible source of health care data, recently spent nearly $7 million to collect signed informed consent from patients residing in a suburban county to satisfy a Minnesota state confidentiality law. Only 24% granted their consent.[8] This low level of response is a bellwether of patient willingness to disclose personal data through one of the most respected healing institutions in the nation. This meager response may erode confidence in the completeness of the Mayo database, but more importantly, it indicates an erosion in the level of trust between a significant number of patients and a well-known provider of high-quality care. If this is a challenge for one of the acknowledged premier clinical care groups in the nation, what insurmountable obstacles might other providers face in the future?

Tough Questions and Dealing with the Details
To make any headway in the debate, patients and healers will need to answer difficult questions in six different areas of privacy, confidentiality and security. These are related to:

- patient consent and authorization
- data collection and use
- data management
- patient rights to view and correct records
- penalties for violations
- federal and state legislative autonomy

The first set of questions relates to the limits of patient consent and authorization: How detailed must the patient's consent be for

---

the disclosure and use of information? Should consent be required each time a patient's data are used, or is a blanket consent for any use adequate? Does it make a difference in granting consent if the patient information is "blinded" so the user does not know the identity of the patient? Should researchers and health plans pay patients for the use of their data? Should patients be required to "opt in" or simply allowed to "opt out" of case management and pharmacy compliance programs?

The second set of questions concerns how the data are collected and used: What data will be collected and how will they be used? What patient identifiers will be used? Will patients be required to consent to the use of their data in return for reimbursement for care? Will every transaction between patients and healers be recorded, even if the patient pays cash for the service? Must patients consent to the use of their medical records for health systems management, public health studies and medical outcomes research? Should law enforcement be allowed to use records for medical fraud or felony investigations? Will pharmacies and case management specialists be allowed to use information to improve compliance and educate patients? Can health insurers use the data to exclude patients with expensive conditions? Can lists of patients be sold to commercial companies for special promotions to patients?

The third set of questions relates to how information will be handled once it is collected: How will data be managed to preserve privacy, confidentiality and security? How long will medical records be maintained? Like certain other records, must they be expunged over time? How can patients be sure that a researcher, or other user of "blind" data, has not merged the data with other data sets that could reveal their identity? Does a patient have a right to privacy on all medical matters, including communicable, fatal and expensive diseases? Must all patient releases be in writing? Once a patient allows his data to be used, how long must confidentiality be maintained? Does it extend after a patient has died? Does the family of a deceased patient have a right to determine whether his data can be used? Can a child be protected against the disclosure of data about a parent, in instances where genetic information could be available and cause harm to the child or other family members? Should patients be required to disclose data as a condition for receiving public or private health insurance coverage?

The fourth set of questions addresses patients' rights to view and correct medical records: Should medical records be like credit records, and should patients have the right to view and correct them? Who will prevail if a patient and a physician disagree on the content of the record? How will patients be allowed access to records? If uncorrected records are shared and the patient later learns of inaccuracies, must corrections be made through the entire chain of data users?

The fifth set of questions involves the penalties that will be imposed for violations: How will intentional and unintentional violations of privacy, confidentiality or security be punished? Are individuals who violate privacy responsible along with their corporate employers? Should those who hold and use data be licensed and periodically inspected? Should data users be subject to criminal background checks?

The final set of questions covers which laws will win in a dispute between the national and state governments on these issues: The federal government is lagging behind the states in setting law, but will federal legislators claim superior jurisdiction and preempt state laws? Should federal laws create a "floor" over which stricter state laws can be imposed? How will conflicts between the state and federal laws be resolved? Which state laws will prevail as health care providers operate across state lines and face different standards in data management? How will internet platforms be subject to state and federal law? If patients voluntarily place their records on internet sites, which rules govern privacy?

Engaging the Covenant
The Congress, the rule-making process and state legislatures are the forums where these privacy matters are already unfolding. They are also the same settings in which efficiency is being debated and demanded. Privacy and efficiency goals require the immediate attention of healers and patients in health care settings, since these are issues that must be engaged between the two most essential parties to the healing—the patient and the healer. Only then can privacy and confidentiality be addressed within public policy settings. Only then can the tradeoff be addressed. Without this step-wise progress, first, between the healer and patient, and later, with others involved in payment and health care policy and management, the trust that is so essential to healing will be substantially eroded.

Medical oaths, as they were initially constructed, could not possibly have envisioned the uses of information and the imperatives of the tradeoffs we face today in modern health care. Only by addressing the issues squarely in the context of the healing relationships and articulating the tradeoffs we face today can we facilitate a public policy resolution. Without such a clear and open dialogue, the healing we seek in caring for patients will be at risk. Patients may become less willing to provide accurate and complete information to their healers and may be less willing to have that data shared for the research purposes that improve care and create efficiencies. The potential to build, or conversely to erode, trust is very great in this aspect of caring and keeping covenants. There are a number of possible avenues for acting within covenants concerning privacy.

Whether in individual clinical encounters, in union contract negotiations, in local town meetings or in contracting with health plans, the issue of tradeoffs between health care cost savings and privacy and confidentiality must get more of the attention it deserves. This is a complex issue that will be worked on for at least another decade, so we may as well start now to work together better. Making that investment in the dialogue will be well worth the time and effort required. There are a number of steps we can and should take immediately.

- Subscribe to the covenant. Privacy, confidentiality and security issues call for the broadest possible recognition among healers of their status within the covenant. This means that not only clinicians, but all those involved in the payment, research, data management and e-commerce businesses using data should subscribe to the same oaths that grew from the sacredness of the healing professions. Whether treating an individual patient, processing a payment claim for a single patient, or researching the patterns of disease for a group of patients, the goal is healing and the adherence to the covenant to serve those patients should be clear and unambiguous. These protections should be subject to laws and regulations to further assure patients.

- Understand the uses of data. Healers who collect information from patients in the course of their work should become better acquainted with the various uses of the data as it flows downstream from their offices. This would include their knowing if insurance claim or patient encounter data is used solely for reimbursement or systems improvement within managed care, or if the data are also to be sold and used for other purposes. It would require that clinicians understand the role of Institutional Review Boards (IRBs) to assure that if records are accessed without consent that confidentiality is protected. This is important for several reasons. First, the knowledge is necessary to fully inform patients how medical records might be used. Second, this understanding is important for assuring the accuracy of the data for potential users downstream. In recent studies of hypothetical patients who needed but could not afford care, significant numbers of physicians were willing to distort the clinical picture in order to secure payment.[9] Would they be so inclined if they knew the data were being used for other purposes in addition to payment? How might such distortions create problems in health services research, physician and patient profiling and government investigations of fraud?

- Maintain privacy and confidentiality and address the tradeoff. Those who are healers have a covenant responsibility to maintain privacy and confidentiality of medical records, to use the information only for healing and to discuss doing so with patients. Those healers, whether they are individual clinicians or third-party payers mining data banks, should inform patients of the important and necessary uses of data for research, public health, disease management and quality monitoring and seek their informed consent. This will lay the groundwork for a patient's own consideration of the trade-offs they are being asked to make. Today's consent forms are inadequate and do not describe the uses or users of a patient's information. Patients are not fully appraised of where, how and by whom their data may be used, and this is a clear violation of the covenant.

- Participate in public policy. Flowing from the covenant with patients is an obligation on the part of healers to address privacy and confidentiality issues in public forums. Whether or not they are engaged in individual patient clinical care, a corporate-structured medical enterprise, or in data man-agement, use and sales, all healers are involved with data, even if all they do is collect it. Public forums are one way to assure that patient stakeholders are involved in making the tradeoffs between the privacy they appear to clearly want and the health economic efficiencies they clearly demand.

- Confront the tradeoffs. Patients, for their part within the covenant, should consider how their escalating demands for more care, more efficiency and more effectiveness are at odds with their simultaneous interests in privacy and confi-dentiality. If it is not possible to "have it all," then what are the priorities? Which of the demands—access, quality, efficiency or privacy—is the most important?

Americans appear to be willing to relinquish privacy in many ways. They do not object to background checks on nannies and child care workers, they use credit cards with impunity knowing that profiles are being created and used and they disclose their unique Social Security number without a thought. But are they willing, as Bernadine Healy, former director of the National Institutes of Health, has asked, to allow the government and others to be trusted with such "sacred secrets" as sexual practices, impotence, abortion, suicide attempts and other "potentially prejudicial" illnesses, procedures and medications?[10]

Is gaining efficiency in health care enough of a reason to allow broader use of medical information? Is detecting fraud so important a goal? Is gaining new knowledge through research a compelling rationale? Is the richness of the available data and the power of technology to use it too appetizing to refuse? Can the covenant between healers and patients be maintained, and even strengthened, while addressing privacy, confidentiality and security of medical information? As in the case of most challenges in the midst of an apparent crisis, there is great opportunity. The covenant can be preserved and enhanced if healers—those in clinical care, health care management, public policy and research—recommit to their obligations, if patients commit to theirs and if both work together to make the tough choices in this emerging health care tradeoff.

Chapter 6

Pain and Suffering

Covenant in Conflict with the Law

We all must die. But that I can save him from days of torture, that is what I feel as my greatest and ever new privilege. Pain is a more terrible lord of mankind than death himself.[1]

Albert Schweitzer

If more people suffered visibly from the pain of terminal illnesses, it would no longer be a hidden issue. Unrelieved pain would not be the unseen killer of the spirit that it is for so many people today. It would no longer test the resolve of the dying to live out the final days of their lives. It would no longer force families to confront the awful choices of the end days, including those choices of assisted suicide.

People today suffer, but they do not suffer visibly. They are most often at home or in nursing homes. Sometimes, but not always, they are in hospice care. At any rate, they are out of sight and out of earshot. They do not grimace as they pass us by in shopping malls, do not cry out at movie theaters, and do not shed their tears getting groceries. They and their families are most often alone and too often isolated, consumed with managing the hour-to-hour torment of unremitting pain along with the other aspects of the terminal disease, its frailties, fractures and bleeding. If those suffering were visible to us, their pain would be front-page news and would be stirring action in larger numbers of important medical and policy centers of the nation. If their caregivers were not so overwhelmed with the task of easing the pain as they supported the dying, they would be organized into effective, policy-changing groups. They would borrow a page from animal rights activist strategies and confront us with our lack of compassion. They would question our humanity toward fellow men and women.

The Extent of Pain in Terminal Illness
The best statistics are on cancer deaths and pain. An estimated

eight million Americans will die from cancer, of whom 70% will have pain and fewer than one-half will be adequately treated for it.[2] Coping with the diagnosis of cancer and adjusting to the shocking news are challenges in the early stage of the disease. Coping with the fears of unrelieved pain comes soon thereafter. Becoming a burden on family members is the principal concern of dying people, and the fear of pain is the next most difficult problem they face. The fear itself even exacerbates physical pain. Unrelieved pain leads to suffering. Cancer is not the only terminal condition that creates pain, but it is the one for which we have the best statistics. Nor is pain associated with only terminal illnesses. Many people who are not terminally ill also experience pain.

In our society, many suffer from other causes of pain and rely—or should be able to rely—on our compassion and care. Chronic pain effects over 50 million Americans and another 23 million experience acute pain from surgery and injuries each year.[3] Back pain affects over 26 million adults and is the leading cause of disability for people under age 45.[4] Arthritis affects one in six Americans,[5] and 23 million suffer from migraine headaches.[6] Pain is estimated to cost $100 billion each year, causing over 150 million days of lost work.[7] A majority of people with pain cannot engage in the normal activities of daily living, such as grocery shopping, walking or housekeeping.[8]

If we as a society are unable to deliver pain relief to the dying, how can we expect to demonstrate compassion to the living? If we are unable to address the clear and unambiguous needs of pain relief in terminal conditions, how can we address those that are chronic? If we are helpless in the face of the conflicts that cripple our compassion in death, how can we expect any better in life? How can we ask those who suffer pain to bear it silently while we discuss public policy conflicts? How can we ask them to suffer endlessly because we cannot resolve our differences about the management of pain? How can we justify our failures when the covenant to relieve the pain of those who are dying should be so clear?

Addressing Pain: A Critical Test of the Covenant
The willingness to address pain should not depend on the visibility or invisibility of those who suffer, the number of people who are suffering at any given time, or what the cause of their suffering might be. Whether they suffer in our midst or alone, they suffer. Whether pain is common or rare, they rely on healers for relief.

There is no place in our healing for judgments about the cause of the nature of their pain. Whether those suffering are children dying from cancer or elderly dying from the effects of life-long cigarette smoking, they need supportive and palliative care. Our healers have a covenant with them to relieve their pain, and our communities share that covenant by assuring that our public policies do not prevent the best possible palliative relief of their symptoms. All are deserving of compassion. Unlike beliefs common in the Middle Ages, pain is no longer viewed by large segments of society and within the healing professions as a signal of divine retribution or a requirement for eventual salvation. Although there are some who value suffering and should be supported in their choice to do so, the vast majority of people today would rather have effective pain relief in order to be better able to put their personal affairs in order at the end of life. Regardless of the nature of their disease, the number who suffer or are isolated in their dying, those who are in pain require care. If that pain is not relieved, it creates suffering, and suffering is another matter altogether.

Beyond Pain: Suffering

The terms "pain" and "suffering" are sometimes used interchangeably, but they are actually quite different. Pain is "an unpleasant sensory and emotional experience associated with actual or potential tissue damage."[9] This can include aching, burning, numbness, loss of sensation, itching and tightness. Suffering is a broader concept and goes beyond the sensations to encompass the hopelessness that some dying persons experience. In suffering, people feel a threat to their existence and to their "integrity as persons."[10] Suffering reaches into the heart of personal, family and spiritual experiences and generates feelings of helplessness as well as hopelessness.

Regardless of how intimately we know a dying person or how remote they may be from our daily lives, the importance of this problem merits more concern. Those who are healthy and active have the means to reach for an analgesic to deaden our ordinary daily pains. Shouldn't we devote a portion of our efforts to helping people in our communities whose pain is more overwhelming and more compelling than our headaches, stiffness and muscle strains? Society should be concerned that people suffer needlessly. Instead, we have made them and the pain in their terminal illnesses invisible and have refused to come to terms with our responsibilities to help.

There are many methods to relieve pain. Some require long-term efforts of caring individuals to teach meditation and relaxation techniques and to assist at the bedside to help patients change positions, remain comfortable, prevent fractures and be free of sores and wounds. Doing this, however, requires time and attention be devoted to these patients. Many people are not inclined or cannot be helpful in this way; few participate as caregivers and volunteers in hospice and respite programs. Although approximately 500,000 patients use hospice services each year and the costs are covered by Medicare, most Medicaid and many private insurers, a recent survey found that only 22% of all families who experienced a terminal illness used hospice services. Sixty percent of those patients had cancer, yet only one-half of all cancer patients used hospice services.[11]

Relieving Pain and Easing Suffering

The easiest and quickest method of relieving pain and easing suffering and demands the least time and attention, involves the use of medication. This method would seem to be best suited to those who cannot or will not take the time for the more personal forms of care that might be effective for many dying patients. Medication also appeals to the quick-fix inclinations and demanding lifestyles of those who are still healthy. Drug methods, however, are precisely at the crux of the controversies in caring for the pain of the terminally ill. Communities have allowed biases about powerful drugs interfere with the relief of soul-crushing pain. Fear of powerful medications interferes with the compassion that should be expressed for the dying.

Ever since soldiers returned from modern-era wars with addictions to the pain-relieving medicines used to treat their physical and emotional wounds, society has become suspect and fearful of the power of legitimate medicines. Solving the problem became the task of law enforcement, which monitored the practices of physicians to assure they were not enabling addicts and creating new ones. These intrusions led to physicians' fears of prescribing these medicines for legitimate purposes and to regulatory barriers to make it more difficult for them to do so.[12] Special prescription pads were needed, special records were kept in pharmacies and forwarded to state authorities and physicians could be questioned at any time about patients who were using these medicines.

Newer, more effective pain-relieving products became available. Physicians were not well educated about them because the legal barriers and risks to using these pharmacotherapeutics were so

---

great that physicians preferred not to use them at all. Why engage in becoming expert in the value and appropriate use of new medicines one would be unlikely to prescribe? Old biases about the nature of the drugs and their effects on patients were therefore left to prevail. Even patients with terminal illnesses feared addictions and many people avoided discussions about pain. Of all the families experiencing a death, only 2% had given any prior consideration to issues involving pain relief.[13]

Everyone—families, patients, physicians and law enforcement—was ill informed and wrong. Patients treated with medications to relieve pain in terminal illness rarely become addicted.[14] Some physicians feared that increasing the dosage to the point necessary to relieve the pain would result in the patient's death. Wrong. Research debunked that theory.[15] Others feared that, left in the hands of patients, overdoses would be common in suicide attempts. Again, the popular notions were wrong; patients would rather live than die.[16] It is the pain they wish to avoid, not life.

Families Seek Better Relief from Pain

The impact of unrelieved pain for patients and the loved ones they leave behind is profound. Only recently have we been able to document that family members giving care to seriously ill or disabled relatives suffer higher rates of mortality.[17] It is one of the most stressful times in family life, and one for which little financial or community support exists. Caregivers, who provide somewhere between $100 billion and $200 billion in uncompensated care, receive few returns from the communities that might otherwise support them with respite and other services.[18]

Beginning in the 1970s, this suffering led to the formation of a number of organizations dedicated to seeking a way out of the fear through political and legal solutions. Unable to find pain relief from healers and incapable of negotiating through the restrictions imposed by law enforcement intrusions into their care, families turned to politicians for intervention.

Their efforts over ten years of working with Congress brought their concerns to a head in 1982, when the National Committee of the Treatment of Intractable Pain succeeded in getting the attention of sufficient members of Congress. They were able to introduce legislation, force hearings and even gain a vote on a bill to change national policy on the treatment of pain in terminal illness. The Compassionate Pain Relief Bill would have legalized heroin for the treatment of pain of the terminally ill and would have required the Department of Health and Human Services to manufacture and distribute it to pharmacies so that it could be prescribed for terminally ill patients with intractable pain. Advocates for the bill argued that on simple humanitarian grounds the pain of terminal illness should be relieved and the dying should not be required to suffer. They pointed to the use of heroin in England, which for one hundred years had provided effective pain relief. They argued that the British model of pain management should be copied because some patients, especially those with terminal cancer, could not be treated effectively with currently available analgesics in the United States.

At the time, the Reagan Administration officially opposed the bill on scientific grounds. Well-controlled clinical trials of the day demonstrated that morphine was just as effective as heroin in pain relief and newer (at the time) and more potent analgesics had become available.

The debate had one positive effect: It exposed the nature of the problem. The dilemma in the United States was not that there were not adequate medicines, but that the way in which physicians managed pain was inadequate. Physicians in this country medicated for pain in a more limited and ineffective way because of their unfounded fears of addiction and well-founded fears of law enforcement intrusions into their practice. With no such fear abroad, physicians in England used more medication more often on a routine schedule intended to anticipate and prevent the recurrence of pain. It was not, in fact, the heroin they used, but the way they used it that made the difference. The patient advocacy groups were right, but for the wrong reason. We needed change in this country, but not in the pharmaceutical arsenal. We needed a change of law and of heart that would allow for the appropriate medications that were already on the shelf.

The Reagan Administration feared that the use of heroin, even in medical circumstances, would signal that its use for other purposes would be tolerated. In addition, it feared that the presence of heroin in communities would increase the rates of pharmacy and drug-seeking crime and cause its diversion into the illegal drug markets. The bill was defeated. Families, desperate for a solution, forced a vote in Congress. There was not yet adequate consensus at the time about the need for a change in pain-management policy, and anti-drug-abuse forces won the debate. This brought defeat to years of effort to create change. However, the effort did not die. The families were effective in setting the stage for more attention focused on the treatment of pain. The Department of Health and Human Services and the American Medical Association embarked on a campaign to educate physicians in practice. These efforts prompted major policy and educational discussions within the clinical community. Have they been successful?

Healers Respond to Patient Needs

Nearly twenty years have passed. In some ways the situation has improved. New research has produced better pain management strategies. Media coverage of pain management has improved. Recognition of pain as a clinical issue has expanded, its own set of side effects and sequelae are understood and pain has been acknowledged in other previously undertreated groups, such as newborns. A number of new pain management societies have formed within the medical profession. Two of the most important groups, the American Academy of Pain Management and the American Pain Society, issued a joint statement recognizing pain relief as an ethical obligation for all health care providers, including for therapies that may hasten death. They concurred that pain is often treated inadequately, despite available medicines.

> Patients, families, caregivers and physicians continue to struggle with the task of caring for the dying and how best to relieve their suffering. The debate on the moral and medical challenges of care for the dying requires a response. That response demands extraordinary efforts to improve end-of-life care and optimal management of pain and suffering. We have the knowledge and ability to deliver skillful and effective control of pain and suffering at the end of life.[19]

The Joint Commission on Accreditation of Healthcare Organizations (JCAHO) escalated the concern for health care facilities on matters of pain. Its new long-term care manual gives residents the right to expect a quick response to reports of pain and calls for statements to be posted in every patient room that notify patients of this right. In JCAHO-accredited facilities, patients are told they can expect that their reports of pain will be believed, that they will be given information about pain relief from concerned staff and that pain will be responded to quickly and effectively. The JCAHO standard recognizes pain as common, as having serious consequences if not relieved and as an important part of the ethical care of patients. It encourages education and involvement of the family.

Some State Medical Boards and legislatures have also recognized the problems of overzealous monitoring of pain medications and have initiated pain study groups and educational efforts. A majority of states already protect physicians from disciplinary, criminal or civil action for prescribing medications to relieve pain through laws, regulations and Medical Board Guidelines.[20] Most recently, the North Carolina Medical Board ruled that physicians will not be subject to disciplinary action, even if the medications they prescribed or administered to relieve a patient's pain hastened death. Ten states have passed legislation protecting medical professionals and family members who prescribed or administered medications for the relief of pain, even if the medications hastened the death of the patient, as long as the intent was not assisted suicide.[21] By 1999, another seven states sought to protect physicians and families and have introduced similar legislation.[22]

Have these efforts been effective? A number of physicians, and a significant number of medical organizations, studied this issue and are on record as agreeing that despite the legal and regulatory protections offered them by their states and Medical Boards, law enforcement still intimidates physicians in their actual practices.[23] Actions, like those of the North Carolina Medical Board, were intended to respond to those physician's concerns. In the words of Hospice for the Carolinas President Judi Lund Person, "I think this is sending a message. What we have all been trying to do is to quell real or perceived fear that if doctors prescribe what they think is enough pain medication, the medical boards may go after them."[24]

Have we gone far enough in reassuring physicians? Can we assure patients that actions such as these will help to relieve the pain of illnesses that devastate their loved ones?

Suffering Continues
The family of William Bergman filed a complaint with the Medical Board of California against his physician after Mr. Bergman's death. The complaint requested that the physician be disciplined for failing to prescribe the medications that would have relieved the lung cancer pain he was suffering as he died in his daughter's home. The Board agreed that the pain management for Beverly Bergman's father was inadequate, but they rejected her request and declined to discipline his physician.

Few families have made such disciplinary requests, but family support and lobbying groups are currently recommending this as a strategy for driving change and so this may well be the harbinger of a new trend in patient and family activism and empowerment. If so, it may also prove to be an unfortunate one.

Physicians practicing today, regardless of whether they are educated and experienced in pain management (and most of them are not), are caught in the middle between drug abuse and pain management tensions. Claims similar to those of the Bergman family were recently successful in Oregon when the Board of Medical Examiners disciplined a physician for grossly undertreating pain in six patients. As a part of the disciplinary action, the physician must complete an extensive educational and counseling program.

Although this will be hailed by some as the right prescription for bringing doctors into the proper practice of pain management, it is not. Healers who fail to act within their oaths and according to the standards of practice should be disciplined, but witch-hunting will not solve the dilemmas we confront in managing tough issues such as pain management, which are more social and legal than they are technical and clinical. Actions such as this, if they are abused, will place healers, patients and families in an increasingly tenuous position. To subject those who prescribe and administer medications to the tensions between law enforcement and medical boards without a community-based policy and political resolution places both the healer and the family at even greater risk. It encourages the physician to abandon the patient altogether. It encourages the family to limit whatever medicines are prescribed. As in ancient days, if physicians are made to walk clinical and regulatory tightropes and risk retribution for their attempt to treat the most needy of the sick and dying, they will be inclined to select their patients carefully. Left with no other choice, they may decline to treat those in greatest need of palliative care. If, at any time, healers might be called to defend their practices to drug enforcement agencies and medical boards—neither of which treat patients and both of which are charged with limiting drug use—they might become reluctant to provide that care. If, at any time, families are questioned about their methods and motives for using medication, they, likewise, will be reluctant to do so. The inevitable result for patients will be the painful deaths so many of them fear.

If these actions become witch-hunts, a cycle of fear will be created and will become even more deeply embedded in the care of the dying. Physicians' fears about prescribing important and necessary medicines would exacerbate the undertreatment of patients' pain, which causes unrelieved pain and in turn creates fear among patients and others who watch them suffer. Fear comes full circle. It is the greatest irony of all when patients suffer because two gifts from the gods—the law and the healing arts—cannot resolve the tensions between them for the benefit of humankind they were intended to serve.

Congress Muddles the Issues

Unfortunately, healing and law enforcement clashes were renewed when Oregon voters sanctioned a law allowing assisted suicide under some circumstances. In 1994, and again in 1997, the voters in that state approved a "Death with Dignity Act," which allowed patients to seek the assistance of physicians to end their lives. Unrelieved pain was one, but by no means the only, aspect of dying that was cited by those who encouraged adoption of the voter referenda.

After Oregon passed the law, the federal Drug Enforcement Administration (DEA) informed physicians in the state that they risked losing their federal license to prescribe controlled substances if they used controlled drugs to assist in a suicide. The letter impacted physician practices and the number of prescriptions for controlled substances declined. Those physician/healers, obviously concerned about the implications of being accused of misusing powerful, pain-relieving medications, wrote fewer prescriptions for pain relievers. However, in June 1998, United States Attorney General Janet Reno issued an opinion that the DEA could not prosecute a physician who acted in compliance with the Oregon Death with Dignity Act. As a result, some members of Congress decided to act, launching another round of volleys in the conflicts over medical use of these medications for the pain of terminal illness.

The first was the Lethal Drug Abuse Prevention Act, introduced by Senator Don Nickles (R-OK) and Representative Henry Hyde (R-IL) in 1998. The act was intended to stem the tide of assisted suicide, fueled not only by the developments in Oregon but also by Dr. Jack Kevorkian's challenges to laws in other states. The act would have given the Department of Justice the authority to review the medical decisions of physicians with regard to prescribing drugs that relieve pain. More than 30 respected national organizations representing physicians, patients, nurses, cancer survivors and pain specialists opposed the legislation. The positive aspects of the bill to improve palliative care were more than undone by the fears that federal investigations would create. As a practical result of the bill, not only would the actions of prescribing physicians be investigated, but the motives of the physician as well. The legal burden of proof, even in a drug abuse–paranoid society, would have remained on the investigators, but the impact on the physician, left to demonstrate that his or her motive for prescribing the medication was not assisted suicide, would have been disruptive to their practice. It was widely feared, and rightly so, that it would have the chilling effect of creating even greater fears among physicians. Those most compassionate and technically competent healers, who chose to stand by and assist dying patients in pain, would most certainly have been at greatest risk.

The legislation died. However, it rose again in 1999 under a new name. The Pain Relief Promotion Act of 1999 retains the essential components of the 1998 proposal. A third bill, the Conquering Pain Act, was introduced in response to the other proposals by Senator Ron Wyden (D-OR) and Senator Connie Mack (R-FL). It improves education, develops community resources for pain management and requires studies to determine how government-funded programs can better manage pain. It calls for a study of pain management by the Institute of Medicine (IOM) a highly respected and visible advisor to government. It will not resolve the problems we have created over the past five decades, but it will be a step in the right direction. The Pain Relief Promotion Act of 1999 passed the House and has been endorsed by a number of clinical groups, pain societies and patient interest groups. It has redeeming features, particularly related to funding authorizations for education in pain control. It also, however, continues to promote the second-guessing of clinical intentions of prescribing physicians. Is it the best step we can take to aid the dying?

Communities in Conflict

At the root of the problem is America's drug abuse problem. We know from public service advertising that drugs fry your brain, and a majority of the kids who use drugs don't live in big cities. Full-page ads tell parents how to talk to their kids about drugs and show them how to plan their child's funeral if they don't. Some employers require pre-employment drug screening; others conduct drug tests on a periodic, and sometimes surprise, basis. Statistics from the Drug Abuse Warning Network (DAWN) report on the level and type of drug abuse activity. Local and state police and the federal DEA arrest dealers and users and display their conquests of these illegal networks with pride. There is no doubt that drugs are a problem that both law enforcement and health care experts need to address.

Preventing and treating drug abuse in this country is a valid objective, but it cannot be the only one. It is necessary, but it is not sufficient. We must also prevent and treat pain in terminal illness, and we know that is a problem for this country as well. It is a part of our lives and of our arts. It is portrayed in *Terms of Endearment* and in the Pulitizer Prize-winning play, *Wit: A Play*. In these portrayals, we, as humans who ought to know better about how to care for each other, do not fare well. We speak, in our culture, as if we care about both the drug abuser and the terminally ill patient, and yet we act as if we care only about one to the exclusion of the other. What happens when law enforcement and medicine are at odds? What happens when they clash? Why is it that when some of us abuse drugs, the rest of us become suspect if we use that same substance for medical reasons? Can we reduce the suspicion about the valid use of medicines to treat pain? Will we ever correct the tragedy of underprescribing the medicines that patients need as they die in pain?

How can we better resolve the tensions between law enforcement and the practice of medicine? How can our communities better balance the need to keep the streets safe from illegal drugs and yet ensure that patients in pain get the medications they need for relief? How can we protect physicians and nurses from harassment and provide patients with medicines while we sort out our differences about drug abuse prosecution and legitimate prescribing? How can we come to agreement more quickly so that more of us do not suffer needlessly as we die?

Confronting the Challenge of Compassion within the Covenant

"Compassion" means "to suffer with," and we do precious little of that in the United States today. Dealing with the pain of some terminal illnesses and relieving suffering at the time of death have been among the most sacred responsibilities of healers for thousands of years. It should be no less the case for us today. In fact, the burden of compassion within the covenant should be even greater because in this era, unlike in earlier times, we have better methods for accomplishing the goal of pain relief. If we apply those methods well, we can assure virtually all patients that virtually all pain can be relieved.

Compassion for the pain of illnesses that cause death should be the hallmark of a civilized society and a central tenet of the healing covenant. In undertreating pain, we do violence to patients at a critical time in their lives. This problem is not a new one and

---

is in no way related to the proliferation of managed care or other reimbursement changes in health care systems. It is, instead, the result of factors that have their roots in denial, ignorance, and conflict—all of which create fear and, in turn, allow pain to rule in the final days of terminal illness for too many people. It is clear that we are at loggerheads in this country on this matter. Law enforcement agencies, and recently some members of Congress, have ignored the very real suffering of the dying. They draw hard lines around the use of pain-relieving drugs and neglect the fact that healing entails the soft side of compassion. Healers, though they have recently become more effective in engaging in the policy debates, remain too silent on the challenges of pain management. We have failed to resolve our differences, and while we are deadlocked in conflict, our dying suffer.

The issues are clear. Should we, as a society, formally invite Congress and law enforcement into the covenant between the dying patient and the healer? How would that be accomplished? What experiences of care-giving would serve to educate them on the realities of pain? What remedies would we ask they pursue if these experiences commit them to caring? Are we asking the dying to disengage from the covenant and suffer because we fear our addictions and doubt our ability to manage them? Are we asking them to suffer in isolation because to see their pain makes our communities wince? How can we balance the needs of our covenant to care for both the dying and the addict? Can we protect healers from bearing the brunt of the conflicts?

Creating a Covenant to Relieve Pain at the End of Life

Today, we have the most extensive arsenal for the management of pain in the history of medicine. No era has had such powerful pain-relieving technologies. Our medicines, surgery and complementary methods of pain relief are more developed now than at any time in history. Our understanding of the nature of the terminal illness and dying process has never been richer. Each pharmaceutical product is researched, manufactured and licensed as safe and effective for working its miracles. Today's methods rarely fall short. Yet no healing responsibility has been so severely tested. Even those within weeks or days of dying are frequently denied the pain-relieving medicines that could ease their suffering, enable them to put their personal and spiritual affairs in order and deal with the grief of their impending death with family and friends.

There are important ways that healers and communities, acting within their covenants with patients, can address these conflicts. The covenant between the healer and the patient was reinvigorated within a new paradigm with the work of Elizabeth Kübler-Ross. The work of Dr. Kübler-Ross brought us a new appreciation for the value of living embodied in dying and showed us ways to support the process of living until the end. That work extended through the hospice movement and has been institutionalized by health care reimbursement, patient demand and volunteer service. Hospice has created a critical mass of patients and healers who, working together, have improved care and pain-management options. They entered into a covenant of obligation. The healer provided the supportive caring of human touch and palliative medical technique. The patient allowed the healer into his personal life, shedding intimate and protective boundaries and disclosing the seriousness of his pain and dependence on others. This covenant has not yet succeeded, however, in achieving a final resolution to the intractable conflicts that leave so many in pain, because communities have not yet been engaged to participate. Communities must now enter into a covenant of obligation with its own who suffer and with the healers who relieve that suffering. A number of additional steps are needed to achieve a resolution.

- Those who work in the fields of cancer care, terminal illness and palliative care are in the best position, because of their knowledge and their standing in their communities, to call communities into a special covenant with the dying. In the style of all covenants, they are the parties who can grant the healing pain relief and who can create the obligations that will sustain the covenant. In the context of their own covenants with the patients they care for, they should lead the way to crafting a solution that can assure pain relief for those who need it.

- Congress and communities, for their part, should engage in this covenant discussion, because it is our conflicting public policy objectives that have created the tensions that have resulted in so much unnecessary pain. This will require an intensified dialogue at national, state and local levels among clinicians, families, law enforcement and policy officials who deal with both concerns—those of drug abuse and those of pain. It will also require extensive education of all parties—and particularly national, state and local law enforcement agencies—about the nature of pain management in terminal illness. Finally, it will call for those of us in communities to trust our healers to practice the arts and skills we have empowered them to use to our benefit. We can no longer explain the lack of compassion for the dying and lack of trust in our healers with fears of addiction and abuse.

- Any individual who holds a position of responsibility in policy, clinical care or law enforcement should be required, as a part of this dialogue, to participate in the care of those who suffer from pain in terminal illness. They should see for themselves what has been hidden. They should learn the value of the medications that have been denied to suffering people. They should understand the consequences of their failure to act quickly.

- Each existing and new legislative initiative or regulatory control to prevent or manage drug abuse must be examined in the context of how best to accomplish not only abuse prevention, but also pain relief.

- The new clinical care groups and study centers, formed in the last several decades to heighten the awareness of pain management and conduct pain research, should be more widely acclaimed for their work.

- The press should heighten the awareness and knowledge of the public and the professions about the availability of safe and effective means of managing pain and should work to dispel the myths that prevent good palliative care for the dying.

- Finally, having addressed the most obvious of pain management issues—that is, the relief of pain in terminal illness—we should turn our attention to the relief of the chronic and sometimes unremitting pain endured by many people in this country and throughout the world. Herein lies an obligation within the covenant for those who are dying. Through their stories and the willingness of their families to address these issues where they cast the sharpest shadows and draw the sharpest lines in public debates, we may accomplish a goal to relieve their pain and those of other dying people like them. Calling us to more compassion, however, may help healers and the nation to deal with the even tougher issues of pain suffered by those who are not terminally ill, and who pose even more difficult questions for medicine and society to grasp.

These are simple steps, but they may be difficult to take. The attitudes of everyone involved have been ingrained through years of practice. The suffering of so many is silent. The denial of death is great. It is a task that must be embraced with even greater energy and attention.

Can it be done? I believe so, and I draw my optimism for the future from my brother, Jim, and his wife Nancy, who for more than 20 years have volunteered their time to a hospice group. Jim wants to write a book. He'd call it, "You *Live*, Until You Die." It comes from his experience of seeing the old and the sick die well, living right up to the last moments. It would be a book of warm, tender and funny stories. He sees people laugh right up to the end. His stories echo the words of one cancer patient who helped us understand the importance of pain management back in the 1980s. She said, "I found that when I didn't have the pain, I could forget I had cancer."[25] As healers and as communities, we should offer that to all our dying patients. To do less is to diminish the living of everyone, especially the ones they leave behind.

Chapter 7

Healing beyond Our Borders

Covenant and Medications for the Global Community

Suffering today is because people are hoarding, not giving, not sharing.[1]

Mother Theresa

Recognizing Need

The world beyond our borders is a globe romanticized by television's Discovery Channel and *National Geographic*. It is a fantasy of *Arabian Nights* and jungle princes cartooned by Disney. It is a world of poetry and adventure tourism.

The developing world is altogether different. It is a nightmare of child labor, child soldiers, starvation, death, slavery and war. It is a world with few hospitals. Clinics are a thirty-mile walk from home. Parasites live in the drinking water. Most people do not have access to health care as we know it. Health care spending may be as low as $10 per person each year—or less—and millions die annually from diseases that could be treated with modern public health measures and medical care. People, especially children, die from pneumonia, malaria, diarrhea, tuberculosis and vaccine-preventable diseases. If they do not die, they may be left orphaned when their parents or grandparents die—11 million are orphaned worldwide from AIDS alone.[2] Blood is not safe from HIV, hepatitis B and C and syphilis contamination. Government corruption is common. Public health and disaster relief systems are stressed beyond capacity.

Some of these developing world diseases do not cross the oceans and continents easily to threaten the United States, but some do. Tuberculosis is one of those diseases, particularly as it becomes increasingly drug resistant. Declared a global health emergency by the World Health Organization (WHO), tuberculosis is spreading around the world at faster rates than public health experts anticipated and at much faster rates than they can control.

Dubbed by the Institute of Tropical Medicine as "The Real Millennium Bug," it is spread easily by coughing. A passenger from the Ukraine recently infected 13 people on a flight from Paris to New York, and a child from the Marshall Islands living in North Dakota infected 56 people at home, school and day care settings.[3] They join the growing number of cases in the United States that are caused by recent arrivals to this country.

Even in the presence of the emergency and global attention, fewer than 20% of people infected with tuberculosis are receiving even basic treatments. Public health experts today estimate that 1.9 billion people currently have active disease, and it spreads to 8 million new people each year. As a result 1.9 million people die annually. Even with newly recommended treatments in place, the next generation of public health experts is predicted to see between 171 million and 249 million new cases of tuberculosis and between 60 million and 90 million deaths from the disease during their careers.[4,5] Future scenarios for a disease so easily transmitted are horrifying.

Reaching Out and Responding

Clean water, sanitation, reliable supplies of food, economic development and democracy would go a long way to improving the lives and preventing the diseases of most of the developing world's population. It would also protect those of us who live in privilege in the developed world.

That is not the only reason to reach out, however. An even better reason is that there are people in poor countries around the world in such need and we should live in covenant with them. They live at levels of poverty and disease unimaginable to even the poorest in this country. It is so shocking, in some cases, that even travelers to those places will forget and deny what they have witnessed, becoming numb to the immense needs once boarding planes for home. As health care practitioners and healing enterprises in the United States, we have the technology, the insight and, occasionally, the will to assist in these ventures. Some healers in this country act within a covenant responsibility to care for others in these distant places. Clinicians spend their vacation time overseas doing surgery and treating patients; medical centers send their consultants, journals and books to mission hospitals that can use them; churches sponsor exchange programs and summer trips abroad for teens to build sanitation systems and shelters to help families. Those in health care cannot do it alone nor do we need to. Tackling immense problems such as these requires the efforts of more than a few.

International aid from North American, European and Japanese governments supports development projects and makes contributions to the improvement of living conditions. Private firms, foundations and service organizations also contribute. For example, The World Bank provides $800 million annually to HIV prevention programs.[6] Private non-health care firms doing business in the developing nations of the world contribute to the economy and to health care as well. ENI, an Italian firm, gave the World Health Organization $750,000 to fight malaria in Azerbaijan. BP Amoco financed child nutrition programs in Vietnam. De Beers contributed $2.7 million to the WHO to fund polio eradication and used its own employees to help in the immunization campaigns. Eskom contributed $5 million to develop a vaccine for AIDS.[7] The Bill and Melinda Gates Foundation contributed $50 million,[8] Ted Turner contributed $28 million,[9] and Rotary International committed $500 million to eradicate polio.[10] The Gates Foundation is also contributing $750 million over five years to other child vaccination programs and $50 million to prevent maternal mortality.[11] Kiwanis International pledged $75 million for salt iodization programs sponsored by the United Nations International Children's Emergency Fund (UNICEF) to prevent the iodine deficiency disorders that impair the mental health of children.[12] There is no tally of the total value of donations such as these, but it is large. Even in the face of expansive philanthropy, the need is still overwhelming—especially for pharmaceuticals.

The World Health Organization estimates that 30% to 50% of the world's population does not have access to the medicines it needs.[13] Recently, attention has been focused on the need for the sophisticated AIDS drugs available in the developed world, but the reality is that even many of the basic vaccines and medicines are unavailable to many people around the world. Developing nations are too poor to purchase them on the world market. The professionals who can prescribe or dispense the products are not accessible in many countries, and the infrastructure to deliver the products to the clinic or hospital sites often does not exist. Roads are not passable. Trucks don't have fuel. Land and water barriers prevent easy passage. Refrigeration is not available for products requiring special handling. Wars and natural disasters interrupt the supply of necessary goods and services.

To assist in meeting the needs for medicines, some very inex-

---

pensive products are made available through loans and purchase programs of the WHO and other international agencies. A number of countries are attempting to develop their own local pharmaceutical industry to manufacture generic products. Some medicines are donated by the research-intensive industry in the United States, Europe and Japan in order to make the most modern medicines available to a wider group of people who need them. As in the case of the total health or economic assistance to the developing world, there is no precise estimate of the volume of this assistance, but it is substantial. Those who donate medicines provide the products and, frequently, the technical assistance to assure their correct usage. Working with not-for-profit agencies, donor companies arrange for shipments of large volumes of products overseas. In some cases they also provide the trucks, pay the import duties and provide the healers in order to get the products to the people. Lately, they also combat the public relations fallout of their well-intentioned efforts.

Healing in the Absence of Explicit Covenants

Healing has always been a risky business. If not tampering with the power of the gods, the healer might have been viewed as bargaining with the devil. Fail to cure and the consequences could be great. Lose a patient in surgery and a doctor could be fined—or worse, could lose a hand. Attempting to provide healing services in the absence of an explicit covenant carries great risks as well. This was true of secular healers in the Middle Ages who practiced medicine without benefit of holy orders. It proved true as well for American pharmaceutical companies who donated products to private relief agencies whose mission it was to bring them to people in need around the world. One particular story is notable and provides a clear example of how the lack of an explicit covenant among all the players involved in the healing process can create problems. This is a story of "good deeds punished." It is a story of the unreasonable and outrageous backlash that can befall a healer who acts in the absence of an explicit covenant with the patients and the communities they seek to heal.

It required hard work and generous effort in 1994 for pharmaceutical company Eli Lilly to donate 25 million doses of Ceclor CD®, a potent antibiotic, to Rwanda to treat the wounds people suffered in that country's civil war.[14] The product was a newer, more potent version of an antibiotic already on the market; but it was not yet approved for sale in the United States; and, therefore, could not be donated to help the people of Rwanda, either. Lilly learned of the need for the drug and recognized that it would be of particular help in treating the machete wounds suffered in the war because the company's research showed it to be particularly well suited for treating skin wounds. The company approached Commissioner of the Food and Drug Administration David Kessler with a request to approve the medicine in order to release it to Rwanda. Dr. Kessler and his team worked around the clock over a weekend to review the company's studies and to release the drug for the donation.[15] Rwandan agencies, hospitals, clinics and ministries of health received the drug from the private relief agencies that partnered with the company in making donations such as this. The result should have been public acclaim for the company, kudos for the quick action of the FDA and international thanks for the generosity of Americans. Instead, anti-industry activists unleashed a public relations disaster on everyone involved.

What went wrong? Eli Lilly believed that since the product was needed and requested, it would be accepted when it arrived and used quickly to help the people in need. The company, which was not interested in public relations coverage, was unprepared for the public relations disaster that followed. It was interested in helping. Should Lilly have been prepared for the backlash? How could it have known that the attempt to do good would be punished in the press? What are the motivations for mounting public attacks on donors of products and services? Is there a way to structure the international relationships to accommodate the objectives of all the parties involved? Who speaks for the patients in poor countries who need but will not receive these medicines unless they are donated? What is the best way to help those patients? Can we come to peace with profit and allow those companies that discover and make these medicines—and make profits on some of them—to give them away without such public relations disasters? How can we encourage, rather than discourage, generosity from a nation and an industry that has produced such abundance? How, in the face of such international need, can we not support the efforts of those who are trying to assist? Could the existence of an explicit covenant have prevented the conflicts that ensued?

Dealing with Public Relations Disasters
In the case of the Lilly donation, the United Nations High Commission for Refugees (UNHCR) miscalculated the flow of Hutus back to Kigali, where the medicine was waiting for them. When

Lilly and the relief organizations learned of this, they attempted to recover the drug supply from the warehouses where it was being stored and to redeploy it to other locations where it could be used. They also offered to provide the country with fresh supplies of medicine, since the first shipments were now close to expiration in the warehouses. Rwandan government authorities blocked those efforts, held the drug until the Ceclor CD® expired and then made claims that Lilly had donated expired drugs. The government's version of the story was published by *Time* magazine, criticizing Lilly and leaving readers with the impression that expired, unnecessary drugs were "dumped" so that the company could enjoy a tax write-off for the donation. In its handling of the story, *Time* blackened the eye of Eli Lilly and similar corporate efforts to assist people and nations in need.[16]

Time was trying to make a point. It was a point that needed making, because in the past there have been problems in donations of all types and from all donor sources. Unfortunately, the magazine selected the wrong example. In the witch-hunt to find and punish an errant healer, the magazine's reports oversimplified the complexity of donations and stimulated unproductive conflicts in the international health community. In doing so, it risked a substantial portion of the donations from the U.S. companies who were swept up in the wake of the Rwandan *cause célèbre*.

Time assumed that only the pharmaceutical company could have been held accountable. It neglected the facts that drugs are donated from a variety of sources for a variety of reasons and may pass through many hands on the way to the patient. Some donations come from pharmaceutical companies directly, but others come from physicians, hospitals, pharmacies, drug wholesalers, churches and individuals. Many donations come from the United States, but they also come from other countries. The donations may come in shipments of drugs and medical supplies, or they may be consolidated with shipments of food, clothing and materials to build homes. The shipments are rarely delivered directly by the groups making the donations. Rather, they are shipped and delivered "in-country" by private groups with experience in managing the complexity of delivering donated goods. Shipments also pass through the hands of local government officials at customs offices and other stops along the delivery route. These stops incur delays and risk diversion into the black market. The private relief agencies generally manage the problems of war-torn areas, the challenges of tribal conflicts and the problems of transport where no roads exist or trucks can travel. They are familiar with these conditions because their local operatives are often native to the country, or are long-standing missionaries with credibility. They have influence in addition to years of experience. Having trouble with a customs official who will not clear a shipment, for example? Then perhaps this official's third-grade teacher, the nun in the religious order partnering to receive the goods, can place a call to him and expedite the clearance. Unable to land a plane in one country? Then arrange with your field operations to land in a neighboring country and truck the materials across the border, where the customs officials are more favorably inclined to let you pass through. Can't donate what the recipient needs, but something else instead? They'll take what you have and use it to barter for something else on the long wish lists they keep. Sometimes that's how it works.

Relief on a Massive Scale
Natural disasters and changes in political systems—such as in the former Soviet Union, Eastern Europe and Africa during the last decade—have escalated the demand for donated products. In the face of growing international needs, the number of relief organizations and donation transactions also are growing. Yet despite the complexity and size of the donation process, the players are independent, autonomous groups and individuals. They include domestic and international, private, not-for-profit relief agencies, foundations, churches, pharmaceutical companies, hospitals, medical schools, pharmacies, wholesalers, governments, shippers, private practitioners and individual citizens. Some of these groups have decades of experience; others are entrepreneurial start-ups, particularly those serving regions of the former Soviet Union. Some groups are large multimillion dollar operations, some are single individuals with not much more than a passion to save their homelands. This group of varied players has no commonly agreed-upon vision, no mission statement, no standard policies and operating procedures, no accountability structure and no ongoing monitoring. They also have no explicit covenant, either with each other or with those they serve. Given the complexity of the operations, the number of transactions involved and the troubled regions of the world served, it should be no surprise that there have been problems.

In recent years, published reports indicated that problems have sometimes occurred with drug donations and that some donations have failed to serve the needs of the organizations and people receiving the products.[17,18,19,20] With increased scrutiny by the WHO and, more recently the U.S. Congress, it would be no surprise if potentially more major crises were to surface. Donors, frequently unfamiliar with local needs and circumstances, have created problems in areas they intended to assist. During the Armenian earthquake in 1988, 5,000 tons of drugs arrived, of which 22% were expired or damaged. In 1989, during the 30-year war of independence in Eritrea, seven truckloads of expired aspirin were received. It took six months to burn. One unsubstantiated report claims that 50% of the drugs entering Albania during the Kosovo refugee crisis were found to be unusable, probably because the products had less than twelve-month dating.[21] Between 1992 and 1996, over 17,000 metric tons of donated drugs to Bosnia and Herzegovina had to be destroyed at a cost of $34 million.[22]

A number of different types of problems have been prevalent in donations: Shipments included expired drugs and drugs had not been requested by the relief agency. When this occurs, local medical teams, who are already stressed with patients and strapped for cash, must arrange for destruction of the products. Drugs not relevant to the diseases in the country have been sent, again creating destruction costs. Drugs have arrived unsorted, poorly labeled or labeled in a language not understood in the country. This makes use of the drugs difficult in what are already difficult treatment situations in field clinics and hospitals. Drugs have been improperly packaged, exposing the drugs to temperatures and moisture that degrades the products and exposes the environment to contamination from the drugs.

These problems have occurred when those involved are well intentioned but ill informed or ill prepared for the tasks of delivering and using the medicines. In some cases, the donors are local church and service groups, unfamiliar with pharmaceuticals, who purchase and collect medicines and treat them like other commodities, ignoring the needs of dating, refrigeration and humidity controls. This also occurs in cases where medical missions are so desperate for any products that they accept whatever is given to maintain any supplies they can and to have pharmaceutical products for bartering other goods. It is also a problem when hospitals, clinics and wholesalers send about-to-expire products in order to make their products available for others in need. Finally, the problem is created by new relief organizations targeting particular war-torn or natural disaster areas of the world, reacting to the crisis needs of the nation but short-cutting the precautions needed for medicines. As a result, countries and clinics receiving the drugs have been left with the results of good intentions and bad operations. This further stresses their already stressful national situations.

Most pharmaceutical companies and relief agencies have policies and procedures that minimize the chance of ill-informed donations. Questionable donations have rarely been traced to particular companies in the past, but U.S.-based companies take the brunt of public outrage resulting from problems, as was the case for Eli Lilly. It is easy for a company to be in the line of fire. Ultimately, donated product is imprinted with the company name. Find a tablet disintegrated, damaged or outdated in warehouses in troubled regions of the world and the only certainty is the name of the manufacturer emblazoned on the product. The others involved in supplying the products more easily escape scrutiny and accountability. Even when companies do not donate the product themselves—as when relief agencies purchase medicines for donation or when hospitals, wholesalers and others donate inventory—companies can be forced to accept responsibility for the final disposition of products that have long since left their control. Finally, companies' philanthropic gestures are drowned by accusations of corporate welfare. Anti-industry activists have claimed that donations are nothing more than inventory dumping in exchange for tax deductions.

Seeking a Solution

It should have been no surprise, then, when in 1995 the WHO, along with a number of international organizations, drafted *Guidelines for Drug Donations*.[23] These guidelines were intended to facilitate the movement of scarce medical supplies to the most needy areas of the globe. The pharmaceutical industry was a significant target for the guidelines. It was also no surprise that the American companies were under the most scrutiny and took the most direct hit.

In draft form the guidelines were widely circulated and adopted by a number of countries to improve the flow of donated medicines into their countries. The guidelines promote four core principles: maximum benefit to the recipient, respect for the wishes and authority of the recipient, uniform standards of drug quality and effective communication between the donor and recipient.

In practice, the guidelines state that

- Donations should be based on need, relevant to the disease pattern of the country and sent only with prior clearance from the recipient, except in emergencies.

- Products should be registered for sale in the recipient country, donated in the formulation and strength similar to those used in the originating country and appear on the WHO Essential Drug List (EDL) or the drug list of the country.

- Products should be from a reliable and quality source, complete with labeling in the language of the country and in large quantities. Products should have at least one year of shelf life upon arrival in the country, unless the recipient knows shorter-dated product is arriving and can properly use it.

- No products should be donated if they have been issued to patients and then returned to the pharmacy (a common practice among European donors), or if they have been given to doctors as free samples (formerly a common practice among U.S. donors, particularly those associated with physician groups).

- Recipient nations are to be informed of all donations, with transportation, port clearance, storage and handling paid by the donor, and the declared value based on the wholesale world-market price.

Developing Covenants

The guidelines were an attempt to solve the problems associated with donations and have resulted in a covenant, of sorts. They could have resulted in a true covenant if all the players in the drug donation process would have been involved in developing them. They were not. Neither the product donors nor many of the relief agencies were involved in the early draft versions. None of the patients were involved either. In fact, the guidelines, when they emerged in draft, came as a complete surprise to most of the American donor companies and relief agencies involved in making and facilitating donations. It is not possible to craft a covenant without the full range of parties involved. Attempting to do so from the start would have required substantially more effort, and it would have been difficult. Defining the nature of a covenant in global ventures will never be easy, but in fact, doing so is essential. The complexity of managing operations such as those embodied in donations across different cultures, languages, medical systems, political boundaries, infrastructures and players makes defining the covenant all the more critical.

The guidelines also could have been more covenantlike if the value of the healing efforts of donations had been acknowledged and if the guidelines had not been used as a weapon of attack against the donors. Instead, the international dialogue required to achieve the resolution was conducted against a backdrop of controversy. After several years of contentious debates, accusations and counteraccusations punctuated by the *Time* story, the guidelines were finalized in 1999 and are now supported by significant parties to the discussions. At long last, the covenant discussions were initiated.

Significant in this resolution was a meeting held at Notre Dame University in 1997, which should stand as a model for covenant development ventures. The Notre Dame meeting was the occasion of the first global, comprehensive and candid public discussion of the issues involved in donations. Recipient countries described the loss of national pride from having to provide care for their countrymen with donated goods and expertise. The WHO noted the problems of donations that did not fit the profile of planned health care needs of the developing world.

The Notre Dame meeting was also the first forum in which pharmaceutical companies disclosed the challenges of dealing with negative publicity. Saddled with the burden of proving that they did not cause donation problems, companies have been forced to conduct their own investigations of frequently unfounded allegations. All too often they have been left to manage the cleanup of negative public opinion. It was in this context that some drug company representatives admitted that under continued, burdensome threats to company operations and image they might consider terminating product donation programs. Workers in the medical mission field acknowledged that this would present a crisis of unimaginable proportions.

The dialogue that took place at Notre Dame changed the landscape of the debate and began the first, tentative steps toward reaching a compromise that would create a true covenant. It was the first time in anyone's recollection that donors, relief agencies, missionaries and recipient countries discussed their common interests. It was the beginning of fruitful discussions about the best methods to manage a global, multiorganizational, multicultural effort in easing suffering and saving lives with donated pharmaceuticals. It was also the catalyst for donor companies and relief agencies to form relationships that improved each of their separate and joint donation operations with refined policies and procedures. But all parties did not yet agree to a covenant, and so, to political observers, the response was predictable. Attacks against industry continued, taking on a different tone. By late 1997 and into 1998, industry critics opened fire in a new direction. This time, they took aim at the tax deductions for donations. They claimed that the deductions were the driving force in company decisions to donate and, in the case of problem shipments of drugs, were examples of corporate welfare gone wrong.

Managing the Domestic Spin

Those who deal in global healing must be prepared for domestic consequences. In the midst of the international debates, claims concerning irresponsible international donations reached the readership of the *New England Journal of Medicine* in a December 1997 Sounding Board article on problems in Bosnia and Herzegovina. The article reported that as much as 50% to 60% of medical supplies sent to Bosnia and Herzegovina between 1992 and 1996 were "useless or unusable." They cited the discovery of World War II medical supplies and expired and inappropriate drugs among the thousands of tons of humanitarian aid deployed to the site. They stated a common view among some groups that the relief effort may have been used to dump outdated supplies.[24]

This article sparked Congressional reaction in January 1998 when Representatives Dennis J. Kucinich (D-OH) and Fortney H. "Pete" Stark (D-CA) requested an Internal Revenue Service (IRS) investigation into drug companies and other medical suppliers whose goods landed in Bosnia and Herzegovina during the crisis. The threatened IRS investigation served as a wake-up call to donor companies, alerting them to the fact that their philanthropy was being questioned. The IRS did not immediately respond to the Stark and Kucinich request for an investigation, but the major U.S. pharmaceutical companies were eventually exonerated. Dr. Philippe Autier, a researcher who examined the drug donation records on site, confirmed that at least the large U.S. pharmaceuticals could not be blamed for the donations. He did eliminate the big companies, such as Eli Lilly, because "big names don't play that game; what can they gain?" Instead, he named direct retailers, consumers, hospitals and charities as the guilty ones.[25]

This wake-up call was not entirely a false alarm, however. Although it appears that no IRS response will come, other actions may result from Capitol Hill initiatives. The House and Senate considered a Joint Resolution, introduced by Kucinich, to adopt the WHO guidelines. The rationale for the resolution is based on a recitation of the type of anti-industry accounts that characterized the initial WHO guidelines document.

Obligations to the World's Needy Patients

Donations of pharmaceutical products and medical supplies—whether they are shipped from surplus inventory or manufactured specifically for donation—are laudable endeavors that are consistent with an American impulse toward philanthropy. But they are also complicated by an interplay of international political agendas and activists. In the wake of antipharmaceutical industry activity at the World Trade Organization meeting in Seattle in late 1999, these activities are likely to intensify. Unfavorable press concerning donations is an international health activist tool to erode the image of the pharmaceutical industry and limit its participation in public policy discussions. The activists condemn Americans and the industry for their donation policies and interests at a time when the industry is also vulnerable to criticism on other fronts at home. This adds to the risks that companies will consider limiting donations altogether, a most unfortunate necessity, should the controversies not be resolved. If donations are to continue, three challenges within the world's health care network must be addressed: (1) marrying donations policy with other international drug policies, (2) the balance of power among the players and (3) international activist incursions into U.S. tax policy. Covenant can be helpful in this regard because covenants can encourage each of the parties to move beyond limited, self-interest agendas.

The first challenge of linking donation policy with other international drug policies is related to the two-fold strategy to make drugs available to more people on the globe. The first component of the strategy is to eliminate, or at least severely limit, intellectual property rights for drug developers. The second is to entrench the WHO Essential Drug List (EDL), which forms the basis for acceptable donated products in the guidelines.

It is well established in the developed world that patents provide the opportunity for drug companies to gain returns from the risks of pharmaceutical research and development. Without the ability to gain a return on investments made to discover a medicine, no private firm would be able to engage in drug development. Those nations with the best patent protection have been the sources of the most innovations for precisely that reason.

While eliminating or limiting patent life, either directly through law, or indirectly by allowing parallel trade, might seem a reasonable short-term solution to the problem of the availability of medicines, it is unwise from several perspectives. First, it will rather quickly limit the supply of new drugs for the entire world coming from research pipelines as companies are no longer able to sustain research costs. Second, it ignores the reality that many of the disease problems of the developing world will not be treated with current medicines. The companies whose resources would be lost to patent infringement are today researching those developing-world diseases most in need of cures, as noted earlier in this chapter. Third, companies have demonstrated in the past several years that, informed of the need for drugs, they will manufacture medicines for the specific needs of the relief agencies.

A much older issue is that of the EDL. First developed in 1977, the EDL was initially intended to reflect a minimum list of medicines that should be available in every country of the world, regardless of the level of poverty. It provided guidance to assist poor countries in purchasing the most cost-effective products. In recent years, however, the EDL has increasingly been promoted as a restrictive formulary and now is used to regulate the movement of donated drugs. Since the guidelines restrict donated drugs to EDL-listed products, the EDL is further entrenched as a normative formulary rather than a "minimum list." Applying EDL restrictions to donated products is a distortion of the intention of the EDL. It unnecessarily limits the availability of products to people who may need them. Strict interpretation of the EDL also restricts U.S. philanthropy, since only older, generic drugs are listed in the EDL, and these drugs are, by-and-large, no longer manufactured by American companies. If a company wishes to exercise its philanthropic intentions—and many do—they, their partners and recipients in the donations must clear special hurdles to send the proprietary, state-of-the-art products that companies produce today. When these hurdles become barriers, they defeat the purpose of the covenant relationships that should be the foundation of the guidelines.[26]

The second donation challenge relates to the fact that donation policy discussions are hampered by an underlying imbalance of power and accountability. This is a covenant issue as well. It is important to resolve this issue of power among the players. Unfortunately for people in need, and wholly inconsistent with a covenant, the guidelines, as they have been implemented, provide a mechanism, to "balance" the power. They give the recipient countries the "power" to refuse donations for downstream users. This has resulted in some unfortunate lost opportunities to provide care to needy people. Medical missions of surgeons, on one-week trips overseas, have been denied entrance at the border because the drugs they were carrying and would use in surgery in the coming week lacked twelve-month dating. In 1998, entire shipments of requested medicines to Haiti, Kenya and Egypt were denied acceptance because a portion of the products had less than twelve-month dating. As a result, the people of these countries did not receive an estimated 200 to 400 cartons of antibiotics, pain relievers and vitamins, among other basic products, due to the strict interpretation of the guidelines.[27]

Additionally, donor companies—usually large pharmaceutical firms in the case of medical supplies—exercise great and independent power because they choose whether or not to donate. Some relief agencies and others purchase the products they donate in the United States or in other markets, but the bulk of donated products comes directly from the manufacturer. The relief agencies that deliver the goods are intermediaries between the companies and the recipient nations. Since the relief agencies are dependent on the companies for products, some of them, particularly the smaller operations, at times feel obligated to take any product, regardless of need, in order to ensure that the pipeline of donations remains open.

On the other hand, some relief agencies exercise power over the recipient governments and clinics that receive products and distribute them to other health care providers or patients. The recipients are wholly dependent on both the companies and relief agencies, and likewise, they must work to maintain good relations with upstream suppliers. Products flow from the companies out to the relief agencies, then to the recipient countries and to health providers and finally to the patients. Consequently, the companies appear to exercise the greatest power in the transactions. As a result, they operate within a covenant of grant. They are, therefore, held to the highest level of accountability among all other players and frequently held accountable for actions over which they have no control. Many donors today, however, are calling for relationships of mutual responsibility and accountability—a covenant of obligation, though they do not use that specific term. In so doing, all parties would work more cooperatively to assure the desired goal. In the course of refining donation operations in recent years, this is beginning to happen. Many of the donors and the larger relief agencies have worked to assure that communications are improved and good records of transactions are kept. As a result, donations have actually increased, even in the face of negative publicity. These policy and procedural changes enhance and operationalize the growing covenantal relationships among the involved groups.

In reality, since donations advance the agendas of all the players, donations should be managed within a set of interdependent relationships bound in healing covenants. It is an optimistic trend that, increasingly, they are. Donors receive the satisfaction of meeting philanthropic objectives, improving corporate image and seeding future markets. Relief agencies meet their organizational missions more efficiently. Recipients care for the needy with the benefits of free, developed-world technologies. The WHO guidelines take some steps in distributing power among the players, but could take more steps to create true accountability and interdependence among them. For example, the guidelines only briefly address the responsibility of the recipient countries to distribute the products efficiently to meet patient needs, but they do not yet require any substantial accountability of the recipients back to the donor through reporting of treatment programs and their impact on health. As these final guidelines are implemented, and in subsequent revisions, new discussions can create a forum among equals in which each party would recognize the value of donations to the others and reach toward mutually beneficial solutions to problems. More relief agencies and recipient countries would then be free to follow the lead of most responsible groups today, who refuse unneeded product without fear that they will lose future donations. Companies, in turn, could require information concerning the use and impact of their donated products and could be better prepared to deal with any negative consequences of the donations.

The third donation challenge relates to the fact that international activists are critical of American tax policy that rewards personal and corporate philanthropy with deductions. As a result of their disagreement with our national policy, they intend to lobby for the elimination of tax benefits for donations—at least for pharmaceutical donations. Non-U.S. players and activists view donations as mere tax strategies, since ours is the only country in the world that encourages private philanthropy through its tax code.

It is unlikely that their efforts will be successful, though any debate could be damaging to the pharmaceutical donation climate. The U.S. Tax Code has supported the deductibility of donations of all sorts since the enactment of the first U.S. Income Tax in 1913, which allowed for deductions for charitable contributions. Through donations, major educational, artistic and charitable ventures have provided services to millions here and abroad. Public support for individual and corporate philanthropy remains high in this country. Not only is there a support for the policy, but there is action as well. Over 75% of all U.S. households donate to charities and, in the past 25 years, the not-for-profit sector in the United States has grown at approximately four times the rate of the economy as a whole. That makes the United States unique in its private approach to giving. Other countries promote care of the poor through direct taxation of corporations and individuals. This difference in national cultures and policies creates suspicion of U.S. companies' motives.[28]

The resolution of this debate will be particularly important given that, in reality, pharmaceutical companies receive tax deduction benefits whether they donate or whether they destroy products in inventory. The exact calculation depends on a number of factors and each situation is unique, but it is fair to say that deductions do not drive the decision to donate. In fact, although the calculation has never been made, it is probably the case that if total costs of donations were tallied, some companies would find that their donations are actually more costly than destruction of the products. This is because companies pay for much of the costs associated with making most of the donations—not only those in their internal operations and recordkeeping, but also those external costs associated with shipping and handling and import duties on donated products. In the final analysis, for some companies the tax deductions may be an incentive to donate, and for most others, deductions merely remove some of the disincentives to becoming involved in this type of philanthropy.

Sustaining the New Covenant
The Notre Dame conference, the guidelines and all the other communications among the participants in the donation of medical products and services are important steps toward developing a global covenant of obligation to care for those in need. Other steps will be necessary to refine the covenant, to further develop the systems to support the caring and to bring other donors to the table. It is critical for the health of people around the world that we continue to reach out to each other to ensure that the flow of devel-

oped-world technology continues and becomes a torrent of giving. It is critical not only for health, but for peace and prosperity globally.

To that end, donations of all types are important and greatly underappreciated for the contributions they make to the lives of people in developing nations. This is especially true for the pharmaceutical products that reach the remotest places and neediest people. Aside from the safe water and environments, food and housing that the developed world can lend, there is no more important, cost-effective donation than that of a medicine to prevent and treat disease.

Working cooperatively with the industry can result in new programs to create solutions to tropical diseases, as recent experience has demonstrated. Merck developed and now donates Mectizan®, which prevents river blindness with only one tablet per patient per year. Over 250 million tablets have been provided to 31 countries in Africa, Latin America and the Middle East.[29] SmithKline Beecham has pledged to donate albendazole for lymphatic filariais, to treat the 120 million people in 73 countries who suffer from that intestinal parasite.[30] The company has committed to continue the donations until this public health problem is solved. GlaxoWellcome has committed to one million courses of treatment with its drug Malarone®, which will cure over 98% of the patients who receive it, to assist in reducing the suffering and death from malaria.[31] Bristol–Myers Squibb has committed $100 million over the next five years in its Secure the Future™ program to find sustainable solutions for HIV/AIDS for women, children and communities in sub-Saharan Africa.[32]

Some of these programs are still too new to quantify. Even donation programs that have been in place for years have never been quantified across the entire donor industry, and full impact is unknown. The types and numbers of donors and relief agencies are so varied that a complete list would be difficult to compile. The evidence of the value of the products is largely anecdotal.

A recent study by Harvard University Professor Michael Reich is a testament to the complexity and the value of even a limited sector of the donation community's effort to get products to people. Even after years of study, this expert in international public health could not quantify the impact of more than a small segment of the donated products.[33] But we do not need to fully quantify the value of the donations to know that philanthropy from the developed world has value.

Few would disagree with the statement that poor nations and

disaster areas have needs that exceed the capacity of local governments and international health agencies, such as the World Health Organization. We know that there are people in need and there are people who are willing to help. The most crucial thing we can do to address these needs now is to return to our values as healers and Americans as we approach the needy of the world. Will we isolate ourselves and refuse to see the needs beyond our own shores? Will we support or hamper the efforts of those who are the donors? Can the philanthropic intentions of companies prevail in the face of international condemnation? If a resurgence of attacks were to occur, would donors decide that destroying products is a better alternative than donating them? Will the public, once they learn that companies are making international donations, force them to redirect drug supplies to the needy population within this country?

Robert Davies, head of the Prince of Wales Foundation, notes that in workshops to teach WHO and other UN officials to work with the private sector, the tensions mount as the teaching proceeds. Frequently, shouting erupts on both sides. Government officials view the private sector with suspicion and see it as corrupt and immoral. Business people view governments as corrupt and inefficient. In fact, the only thing they agree about is each other's corruption.[34] Coming to peace across the public-private table will not be easy, but it must be done. Coming to peace with the presence of a for-profit sector within the global health care enterprise, likewise, will be fraught with challenge. Lives are at stake as we debate. Coming to peace will involve engaging new partners and learning new skills. Coming to peace will require developing new operations and elevating the concerns for health care in the developing world at a time when America is struggling with its own health care crises. The most recent set of revised guidelines are a start, but more steps must be taken by all parties in order to secure even more comprehensive standards.

This will not happen unless policy and donor players in the United States continue to manage the challenges that still exist in donations and the controversies that may yet occur at home and abroad. If the donation effort a decade from now has survived and grown, those people will be the ones to be thanked. To help them, national policymakers should allocate some time to engaging in the substantial additional dialogue that will be required among the WHO staff, U.S. Congressional staff and members, pharmaceutical companies, recipient agencies, nations and activists.

Some of these discussions might address questions such as:

- Who should take the lead in ensuring the quality of donations? Should it be pharmaceutical companies themselves, who have so far borne the burden of bad press? To keep the donated medicines pipeline open to developing nations, companies should maintain impeccable donation operations, select relief agencies carefully and respond to the political backlash that some donations will likely create. Whether for commercial, philanthropic or image objectives, no company donating medicines today can ignore either its own operations or those of others who may be handling, receiving and even donating their products. Goodwill can be generated through targeted and controlled donations; disasters can be created out of unmanaged philanthropy. The reality is that when donations go bad, it is the company that takes the heat. Should that be the case, or is the donation effort ready for shared responsibility and should others also be accountable on the world stage?

- Who should develop and manage the complex infrastructure required to ensure the quality of shipments under these most extreme circumstances? With a worldwide enterprise at least as large as any Fortune 100 corporation (in terms of transactions, international regulation, staffing, budgets and volume), it is unwise to assume that donations can be managed with anything less than a common mission statement, operating procedures, extensive communications and accountability. Perhaps common sets of forms, policies and procedures should be developed across the entire supply chain, modeled after those used by large, sophisticated and accountable relief agencies today.

- How should the responsible donors, recipient countries and agencies make the effort to eliminate the (usually) smaller, local, irresponsible players in donations, who through their efforts disrupt the internal health care operations of the recipients? Though well meaning, they are uninformed and uneducated in the policies and procedures that guide good donation practices. Their misadventures threaten the entire legitimate donation effort of the responsible players.

- How can non-health care players be brought into the discussions of health care needs to support infrastructure development? As companies like IBM, Dell, AT&T, Healtheon and Microsoft are entering the American health care market, should they be invited into the global donation effort? How can those in the fields of education, communications and economic development be engaged for the good of people's health? Where can their resources be spent to improve the living and working conditions of the local employees? What are the best incentives local governments can provide to increase their involvement?

- Can we bring an end to demonizing profit in the health care sector? Is the greed we perceive just a misunderstanding of the commercial imperatives of businesses that rely on private sources of capital? Is there an alternative to current revenues that will pay for research, or can we come to terms with the need for profit? Do governments want to increase their own levels of research effort to discover the drugs for the developing world, or should companies be allowed to proceed? How can local generic industries be developed to expand the availability of important products without harming progress toward innovation worldwide? How can we recognize that differential pricing in products actually supports access to medicines and that a single worldwide price would spell disaster for all nations?

- Can we stop demonizing government regulators and bureaucrats? Is the inefficiency we perceive just a misunderstanding of their operating constraints? How can those in the for-profit sector support the imperatives of governments? How can the public and private sectors work together to meet their mutual goals of providing care to the needy?

- How can the parties to this debate best understand each other's separate agendas? Can we develop a global research agenda that, coupled with incentives for public and private sectors, could result in new solutions to tropical diseases? Can we find our way through issues as complex as this in a nation (the U.S.) that is currently isolationist in the safety of the post–Cold War era?

In the end, the enemy is disease, not the parties of the debate. The weapons will be cures, not rhetoric. Maintaining the covenants that supply donated products and services and creating new covenants of obligation will require that the most powerful player in the process of drug donations—the American pharmaceutical industry—bear the lion's share of the effort. It will require that the industry work to ensure quality donations through its own donation channels and through the contacts of others, that it weather the storms of public image attacks and that it continue to offer a wealth of products and talent to the developing world. It will not be easy. But it will, in the end, be the single best way for the industry, and this country, to reach out to others on the planet, demonstrate leadership, protect health at home and avoid health isolationist policies that are unworthy of a nation so rich in resources.

Part 3
HEALING HEALTH CARE

In some ways healing has changed substantially since healers first created covenants. Healers today have greater capabilities due to substantial improvements in education and highly evolved diagnostic and healing tools in their armamentarium, as well as the number and types of healers—at least in the way I define them—practicing the healing arts. Today, healers are not just the traditional physicians, surgeons and pharmacists of ancient times, nor are they the allied health professionals who readily come to mind. Healers are all those who touch the health care enterprise. This includes those who manage health information on the worldwide web, develop and market health care products, regulate the health care industry, advertise health care products and most important, control the access and reimbursement streams that fuel patient care.

In at least one significant way, however, nothing has changed. Although the relationships between patients and their healers are in tremendous flux, patients still expect today's healers to act within the covenant to which they have ascribed for thousands of years. Many healers are willing to do so and hold dearly to their obligations despite mounting pressures of practice. For these healers, their patients and communities, steps to reinvigorate existing covenants and create new covenants of obligation may well be the most productive steps to take in assuring a healing enterprise for the future.

If health care is healed, it will be because healers continue to embrace covenants. If health care is healed, it will be because healers call today's patients and communities into new covenants of caring. If health care is healed, it will be because patients and communities responded. If health care is healed, new covenants of obligation will serve as the foundation of the healing enterprise for generations to come.

Chapter 8

Emerging Models

Healing within Covenants

> *Noisy, curious healers who make house calls will have the time of their lives!*[1]

Patch Adams, M.D.

Practicing in New Covenants

Covenant does not require healers to make house calls. But those healers I know working within the emerging covenant relationships evolving today do have the "time of their lives." Perhaps that is why not only their "patients," but they themselves, thrive and enjoy such longevity. I met Patch Adams. I was his patient and so I feel qualified to talk on his behalf. Patch Adams describes his approach in *Gesundheit! Bringing Good Health to You, the Medical System, and Society Through Physician Service, Complementary Therapies, Humor and Joy,* and I know it's for real.

It wasn't a house call. I met Dr. Patch Adams at National Airport in Washington, D.C. in the fall of 1992. It was an early Friday evening and I was waiting to board a flight for home after a long week's work on the road: tired from travel, stressed from meetings and very much in need of a vacation. I was seated at the boarding gate waiting for the flight, when I glanced over my shoulder and saw a very tall, strange character coming through the metal detector. He was dressed more outrageously than any portrayal Robin Williams ever managed in the film version of Dr. Adams' life—a rubber chicken, immense floppy shoes, ballooned pantaloons and a huge nose stand out most clearly in my memory. He was accompanied by a tall woman who was also dressed to draw attention—a cross between Olive Oil, Raggedy Ann and Minnie Pearl. He must have sensed the tension in my executive life from across the room. He headed straight for the seat next to me. For nearly 45 minutes as we awaited the flight's departure for Newark, he teased, he played, he offered a lollipop. He made whistle and hum sounds, but he never spoke. He answered none of my questions, but he engaged me in his brand of healing, delightfully. Having no idea who he was or what this was about, I was polite, but also afraid, amused, and curious. Mostly, I laughed—apparently the medicine he was prescribing. I noticed others in the gate area, they kept their distance, but they watched all the while. They also laughed. Perhaps this was Dr. Adams' view of public health. Not only did he cure me of the fatigue of the moment, but he helped the whole group. I took the lollipop to be polite, but never ate it, for the obvious reason that I suspected it contained a substance that precipitated his unusual behavior. Until the movie "trailers" for Patch Adams arrived in theaters, it did not occur to me that he was a physician, acting as a healer within the covenant he defines, healing everywhere he goes.

Not all of the extraordinary healers I know have articulated their missions or expressed them as outrageously or as well as Dr. Patch Adams, but some of them have. Few of them have published their views and even fewer are known by the public-at-large. None of them are likely to appear on the silver screen, so they are largely unsung heroes except within the spheres of health care where only close colleagues and friends know their work. Although those healers have not embraced a formal covenant, they have acted within one. Although they might not choose to portray their life's work as having been conducted within the covenants of obligation that I propose, I believe they would see themselves in the stories I tell about them and others who work within covenant. None have ever specifically mentioned covenant in their work, their writings or their talks, but they act as if notions of covenant were central to their own personal, organizing principles.

These healers share a number of characteristics in common with Patch Adams, and since his life and views are the best known of those contemporary covenant healers, it tells the story of the others. Like Dr. Adams, these healers look beyond the mechanics of the physical body into a wider array of needs the people they serve have—be they a patient ill with some malady or a healthy person avoiding sickness or improving their fitness. Like Patch Adams, they prefer preventing illness and supporting health over crisis management of illness and disability. They have passion for what they do in caring for others and they are always striving to do it better. They don't dress in red rubber noses, but they have taken risks to engage the resources they needed to create successful practices, as Dr. Adams did. They haven't all defied the institutions of health care and its bureaucracies, but most of them have, and all of them have been willing to engage in nontraditional ventures to accomplish their mission. Like Dr. Adams, they are scholars in their own fields, but they never shied from the opportunity to learn from others or to integrate learned approaches from other fields. They work in teams, and they inspire leadership. Acting as leaders, they have invited others into the covenant, whether as patients, as customers, as employees or as colleagues. They took fewer vacations than they needed, and they were certainly tired at times, but none of them burned out. They have worked long past retirement age or "retired" into other healing ventures. And like Patch Adams, Dr. Gesundheit himself, they are strong personalities and a pleasure to be with.

Healers and Their Emerging Covenants

Covenant pioneers in contemporary healing go beyond good customer service. Their intention is not to grow market share or to limit health care utilization, though those outcomes are frequently the result. It is unlikely that they are known to each other, as there is no trade association or professional society that embraces those who feel the pull of covenant to guide their endeavors. Their stories are largely anecdotal, as few studies have been undertaken to develop a comprehensive picture of what their practices contribute to health and healing. Nonetheless, their contributions are real and important for sharing. Their covenants are implicit, because few explicit covenants have been written. Today's health policy climate is conflict-ridden and anger is frequently directed at healers. Leaders in health care are too often criticized for not having easy answers to tough questions. In an attempt to heal health care, those innovators who are striving to be healers of patients, communities and other healers deserve some recognition and continued encouragement for their efforts.

Some of these healers are professionals we do not traditionally view as being within the healing enterprise. One that comes to mind is an advertising executive, Gil Bashe.[2] His early life experience as a medic in the Israeli army gave him an appreciation for the needs of patients and the importance of nurturing them that translates into a passion for communicating health issues in a way that improves patient knowledge and thus their health. He tells stories about how soldiers in the Israeli army, tough as they come, would need caring when they were ill with relatively simple conditions. He tells an even more compelling story about how he, with the help of others in his unit, cared for a young enemy Syrian soldier in battle, dragging him off the field under cover and treating him for what was already a partial amputation of his leg. Gil says, "There are many ways to communicate and even in the presence of an enemy unit and unable to understand the language, we could see the spark in this soldier's eye that he understood we would care for him. Providing care for him was life-giving for us as well as for him." Gil's mission is to make communications as much a part of life-giving care as the other therapies that healers employ. He wants information, itself, to be healing.

Others are following in Bashe's footsteps. Brother and sister team Julie and Paul Lerner developed and published a guide to health care services in New York, in response to problems Julie encountered during her experience with non-Hodgkin's lymphoma. They work with other patient groups, encouraging them to demand more information, compassionate care and less bureaucratic relationships with payers. They use information as tools of empowerment into the hands of other patients.

Similar ventures are underway through the internet and are now too numerous to mention. Unfortunately, though many sites would claim to be covenantal, not all of these ventures are. Some contain inaccurate and biased information and masquerade as legitimate sources of valid clinical information. Few sites are monitored for quality, and only recently have e-health commerce groups met to form standards of performance that characterize a covenant with patients and communities. One notable exception is the design of Dr. Joe Prendergast.[3] It is called DiabetesWell and it provides a web-based site for information on diabetes that includes quarterly patient assessments, counseling and recommendations for diet, medication and exercise. Patient test data are collected and monitored by the site, which is staffed by Prendergast and a staff of physicians and nurse specialists. New research and information is provided to patients through daily e-mails designed to be read in one minute. True to the nature of monitoring quality in the covenant, Dr. Prendergast tracks the impact of his e-care on patients. Rates of hospital admissions and deaths from diabetes are substantially reduced in his subscribers.

Other covenant pioneers are business executives. Matt Emmens had such passion for healing potential that he left the comfort of a good, secure job to risk it all in a start-up company. That company became the platform for one of the largest pharmaceutical research companies in the world today. Des Cummings created a new health care system, based on new paradigms, in a new town. Des and Matt worked together to fund and launch the search for innovative solutions in health care. They called it the Center for Health Futures, and its work is to link traditional healers with other healers and communities.

Business executive Pat Charmel was profiled in *Inc.* magazine as a hands-on hospital CEO.[4] Griffin Hospital, which he heads, embarked on a multiyear project to satisfy its customers. In the midst of reimbursement rate slashes, revenue declines and competitive consolidation, this community hospital challenged the impossible—to "just say yes" to whatever would satisfy their patients. What the hospital team did was characteristic of covenant relationships, they listened. Sometimes this meant listening to each other as they detailed the bad experiences they or family members had in hospitals. They posed as patients to see what patient care was like at other institutions thought to be "better." It also meant listening to their own patients. Then it meant changing their directions, their procedures, even their bathtubs, if that would satisfy patients. It meant creating community access to the world-wide web for research, visits by therapy dogs and places to bake cookies in the oncology unit. It also meant forcing changes, changes that were not always well received at first. But eventually staff turnover slowed, staff designed even more responsive programs, occupancy is up and 400 community volunteers provide for any service patients need at the moment—including for one patient, seeing that income tax forms left in the car got mailed on time.

Some new covenant healers have personal experience with disease. If they do, they tend to become organizers. Charles (Charlie) B. Inlander and Abbey Meyers created separate venues for patients to act collectively and have a voice in their personal care. In each of their organizations, they have created mutually supportive covenants with patients, and together they challenge healers. Corporations are also healers. CVS, the largest pharmacy in the nation, has invited customers into a covenant regarding medication safety.[5] The company encourages its patients to provide complete information to its pharmacists about their prescriptions, over-the-counter drugs, vitamins, minerals, nutraceuticals and herbal medicines they are taking. In an atmosphere of assured confidentiality, CVS pharmacists can caution against the negative effects that some combinations are known to cause. Other healers support the health policy process. Judy Miller Jones has nurtured the nation's national policy wonks since the Carter era, creating a cadre of reciprocal relationships with them and enabling those relationships, all for the benefit of improving the quality of health policy analysis and decision making.

Researchers like Dr. P. Roy Vagelos are covenant healers. His passion for patients and the mechanisms of disease led him to ground-breaking ideas in drug development and stirred him to challenge other physicians in the way they managed disease. Roy was unusual as a researcher in the days when he explored the healing potential of research. First, he worked as a researcher for a pharmaceutical company at a time when researchers shunned the industry, fearing that working for a company would damage their careers. Roy put those fears aside. Then, he developed the business and management skills needed to turn the labs and clinics into highly successful discovery centers, beating the odds in discovering and developing more drugs than other companies in the industry. Finally, he translated all of those skills into not only managing the internal vision of the company, but communicating that vision through tough times weathered by the industry when the capital markets were losing confidence and investors were leaving biomedicine in droves. He held prices at or below the consumer price index long before other companies followed suit, and he made a valuable parasitic medicine available at no cost to the people of the developing world who could not afford it. He retired to devote his experience to education, new research ventures and philanthropy.

Maurice R. Hilleman, Ph.D., broke through barriers and plunged into a field that was highly controversial—vaccines—and brought prevention to the world's children. He pioneered vaccine research in children and was one of the first to address the ethical issues of informed parent consent and community concurrence with studies of vaccines. Visiting local neighborhoods, community leaders and churches in the Philadelphia area, Dr. Hilleman worked through the concerns about vaccine research and produced some of the most valuable vaccine products available today. One vaccine alone, the Measles-Mumps-Rubella vaccine, which he developed, in part, through throat cultures from his own daughter Jeryl Lynn's illness, is estimated to save the nation $5 billion in direct and indirect medical costs for each birth cohort that is vaccinated. He might have retired long ago, but he has not. Instead, he has continued his research and to advise others in his field of expertise.

Two individuals are unique in their ability to walk both the trenches and the hallowed halls of public health. They have cared for patients individually and have mastered the politics of caring for them as populations. Dr. Bill Foege is one of the most notable of this group for his role in eradicating smallpox from the globe. Medicine and peace are a style inimitable to Dr. Foege in all of his work. He traveled in West Africa in the midst of a smallpox out-break without enough vaccine to immunize everyone at risk. He developed new strategies to contain the disease in Africa and other parts of the world and convinced government health officials to try his radical approaches. He worked in war-torn zones to do it and was held at gunpoint by rebels and in detention twice.

When he returned to the United States, Dr. Foege was appointed to head the Centers for Disease Control and Prevention at a time when it was reeling from the ill-effects of the Swine Flu Immunization campaign and reports of Guillain-Barre Syndrome supposedly caused by the vaccine. He repaired the image of the agency and restored the trust of the nation in its programs and policies, in time to confront a growing number of public health crises: toxic shock syndrome, vaccine safety, Reye's syndrome and HIV/AIDS.

Dr. Foege's experiences and skills are similar to those of the soft-spoken medical missionary Sister Maura O'Donohue, M.D., a physician who practiced for fourteen years in Ethiopia during the wars, and for nine years on HIV/AIDS in the developing world. Like Bill Foege, Sister Maura walks the halls of power where she articulates the needs of her patients well. Some healers practicing in war-torn, famine-struck regions are more at home in their field clinics than in policy and political settings. Sister Maura, a rare breed among them, is facile in both. Her political skills promote the true changes that global institutions must make to save lives. Like Bill Foege, her efforts have resulted in negotiated solutions to glob-al problems of death from disease and malnutrition.

A few pioneers in healing today have crafted the reciprocal relationships central to a covenant of obligation; they are teaching this way of healing to other healers and evaluating and publishing the results of these ventures. As healers, they have proposed new relationships to their patients and their patients have accepted the offer. And now, the healers and the patients are in a reciprocal endeavor participating in and generating the outcomes of cova-nental healing approaches. The list of all those who have engaged covenant, though not specifically saying so, could fill a book. Knowing more about these and others who have approached

healing with such respect could create models for others who follow them into much more demanding territory to address many
more challenging problems in the new millennium.

Over time, these relationships have evolved and are still evolving—neither healer nor patient at this point can say where the relationship will lead. As a result, a significant challenge awaits these
healers, the systems within which they work and the health payers
and policymakers who shape them all. The challenge will be to
assure that, over time, the regulatory and payment environments
don't get in the way. Today's regulated health care is so con-
strained that the sacredness of these relationships is endangered.
New regulatory and payment environments must keep pace with
these changes, allow for the growing covenant-style care and not
"lock in" noncovenant systems of management. The complexity of
the regulations that guide the practice of healing and the reimbursement, as Uwe Reinhardt has said, can make "a crook" of
anyone in health care.[6] It would be a tragedy if those involved in
returning to the roots of caring were prevented from doing so. It is
critical, then, that those regulators and legislators who frame the
legal structure for payment examine their own role in healing and
enter into the covenant accordingly.

Cooperative Health Care Clinics: A Covenant between Patients and Healers

The Cooperative Health Care Clinic (CHCC)[7] is one of the programs worthy of protecting against rigid systems of payment and
regulation. It is an innovative model in which care is provided to
older patients by a team composed of a physician, nurse, pharmacist and other healers in a group setting. It was developed by
John Scott, M.D. and colleagues with funding from Kaiser
Permanente and first piloted within the Kaiser plan. Based on findings from research conducted to date, the CHCC is a cost-effective
delivery style that helps physicians and health care plan administrators improve the quality of care provided to older adults with
multiple disease conditions.

The CHCC model addresses one of the major challenges of
health care today—that physicians' time spent on direct patient
care has been seriously eroded by various mandates of managed
care. In the CHCC model, groups of fifteen to twenty patients meet
monthly in an "expanded doctor's office visit" that includes care
delivery, education, social time and a question-and-answer session. Patients or their physicians have the option to request time for

private visits following the group session, if either should feel the need. In the traditional way that we speak about health care today, we would say that the CHCC model encourages patients to be active participants in the management of their health care rather than dependent recipients of care. In the language of covenants, the CHCC model moves beyond the usual covenant of grant and encourages several types of covenants of obligation between the healers and the patients; first, between the patients within the group; second, between the healers in the group; and third, between the patients and healers together. By all accounts, both the healers and the patients who participate in this form of care are living up to their obligations. They attend the meetings regularly and provide continuing support to each other and their families, including when their conditions cause hospitalizations or death. No study has yet been completed to capture the richness of the relationships, but they are clear from observing the groups in action, from the anecdotes provided by all the participants— patients as well as healers—and from the outcomes measured in the participants in the project.

The initial CHCC program was a one-year, randomized, controlled study funded by Kaiser Permanente and included about three hundred patients. The promising findings of the first study attracted the attention of the Robert Wood Johnson Foundation, which subsequently funded a larger study of eight hundred patients. In both of these studies, the experimental groups attended CHCC sessions and control groups received traditional primary care. The results were favorable. The participating patients showed improvement in their ability to manage activities of daily living, improvement in patient satisfaction, 20%–30% decrease in hospitalization, more than 20% decrease in emergency room use and a decrease in nursing home referrals. Patients liked this care model so much that they stayed with the health plan. Even physician satisfaction was improved, so much so that some of them said they would never again want to practice any other way.

The economic analyses conducted by the CHCC are preliminary, but it appears that among these very old and frail patients, savings have been approximately $3 per member per month. Economists are in the process of applying these findings to a broader spectrum of patients, as defined by diagnosis, health status and utilization. Savings for a broader and largely healthier group of patients are anticipated to be in the range of $50 per member per month. Currently, there are great expectations and significant planning efforts associated with the future of the CHCC. Kaiser Permanente has a goal to establish 100 CHCC groups of 20 individuals for 2,000 of its most needy enrollees.

Covenants with the Uninsured

There is no more challenging issue in health care politics today than how to deal with the growing problem of the uninsured. Those who lack insurance because small business employers cannot obtain or afford coverage for their employees, those who earn too much to qualify for low-income programs and those who are too young for Medicare are a growing segment of those who need care and the funds to finance it. Providing insurance to the uninsured was only partially resolved in programs of the last few decades. Policymakers and politicians have yet to resolve the issue by crafting a final solution that will have sufficient support for enactment into law. Burdened by other patient rights proposals, including proposals to give patients the right to sue for denials of care, some employers predict that their continuing coverage of health benefits is in jeopardy. The number of uninsured may be destined to grow.

A number of communities, in meeting their part of the covenant, have designed programs to provide managed care for the uninsured. The Center for Studying Health System Change is tracking 12 communities intensively.[8] In each case, the community is attempting to provide for primary and preventive care, while avoiding the expensive inpatient and emergency care that sometimes results from a failure to prevent and treat conditions early. These communities use existing charity care funding, Disproportionate Share Hospital (DSH) funding and local tax revenues to provide access to managed care for those who are not eligible for other publicly funded programs like Medicare and Medicaid. They do not provide the identical benefit package as those in entitlement programs, but actively monitor and transfer the patients to public programs when they become eligible. They use a variety of strategies to control costs, including physician primary care managers, provider networks, 24-hour help lines to divert patients from unnecessary emergency room visits, social services, language translators and low-cost transportation to health care facilities.

A project funded by the Robert Wood Johnson Foundation called "Reach Out: Physicians' Initiative to Expand Care to Underserved Americans" has modeled the provision of care for the uninsured through networks of volunteer physicians.[9] Medical societies, group practices, not-for-profit groups and religious organizations sponsored projects to increase access to care, under the leadership of physicians in local communities who recruited and organized participation. Development grants from the Foundation supported the organization of the care, which was provided in freestanding clinics, referral networks, primary care networks and public-private partnerships for primary and surgical care. Approximately 11,000 physicians provided care to nearly 200,000 patients during the four years of the program and, because the projects have demonstrated their value, more than three-quarters are expected to receive local support to continue now that the grant funding period has ended.

Nursing Center concepts have developed out of advanced nursing practices that originated in 1965 and provided general primary care, as well as special care in schools and in nurse-midwifery, in areas where physician care was unavailable and insurance unaffordable. Of patients in nurse practices, 20%–50% are uninsured. They tend to see their nurse practitioners somewhat more often, but use hospital and emergency care less frequently. In some cases these practice arrangements are collaborative with physicians, in others they are independent practices that are fully managed and supervised by nurses, and in half of the states today, nurses can provide primary care and prescribe medications without the supervision of physicians or without collaborative agreements with them.[10]

In an effort to use information technology, the Greater New York Hospital Association (GNYHA) is in the process of developing a system called the Health Insurance Training and Education (HITE) Network, to inform New York's nearly 3 million uninsured about the resources available for their care.[11] In this project, these people will be linked with a variety of resources that are already available, but underutilized. Concerned for the growing number of uninsured, as well as for the number who are eligible for services but not accessing those services, HITE assumes that these individuals are unaware of the resources and simply need to be linked with them. Services such as health insurance subsidies, breast cancer screening, HIV testing, flu shots, free medications and low-cost care will be made known through outreach and information using a web site containing state-specific resources and trained personnel to help uninsured individuals access the information.

In a radically different model, and one that addresses the

affordability problems of the uninsured and the underinsured, the American Association of Patients and Providers (AAPP) has established SimpleCare.[12] The program is built on the vision of both traditional healers such as Doctors of Medicine and Osteopathy, Chiropractors, Podiatrists and others considered alternative or complementary healers, such as massage therapists, acupuncturists, nurses and physicians assistants working together with patients. The AAPP recognizes that each of these healers offers a unique perspective and can help the patient in need, and that they can coexist when patients are allowed to choose their healers. Its goal is to return to a simple system of health care, avoiding the administrative expense and paperwork burdens that have so confused patients and drained the resources of healers. In the SimpleCare program, patients pay for services at the time of the visit in cash, by check or charge card, at a rate reduced from most third-party visits, usually 35%–50% less. The healer does not bill the insurance company, nor provide information to allow the patient to file claims. For uninsured patients who cannot afford the care, some communities have bartering options in which patients can "pay back" their health care costs by providing services to others in the community. The AAPP is not the only such discount program, North American Care operates a similar program, with discounts of 20%–70% for cash up front.

Celebration Health: A Covenant between Healers and Communities
Healers and their communities are also pioneering covenants as communities are becoming increasingly receptive to new relationships with healers,[13] and as community leaders become aware of the roles they can play to support health and healing within their official roles. In one recent study of community attitudes, it was clear that community views of health and healing are ready for new, broader definitions of health and covenants of obligation. Definitions of health are moving away from the avoidance of disease and toward the active pursuit of wellness and an appreciation for the nonmedical quality of life factors in communities. People are discouraged with the health of their own communities, lack confidence in their leaders and institutions and are ready to play a more active role to improve health. Health care reform is viewed as an individual as well as a national responsibility, and a majority of people now believe that they can help by becoming more focused on prevention and on cost-conscious buying of health care services. Declining moral values and selfishness are

viewed as barriers to improvements in health, and the definitions of a healthy community have become more comprehensive. Communities perceive themselves as healthy when the crime rate is low; when they can raise their children in a good place; when children's needs are addressed, including child abuse, child care and education; and where strong family life, positive race relations and affordable housing is predominant. The usual measures health care has come to be concerned about—access, quality and affordability—were considered critical determinants of health for only slightly more than half of the people surveyed. Communities are looking beyond the clinical offices and institutions that deliver care.[14]

It was into that community reality that Disney and its fantasy-world designers stepped when building the twenty-first-century town of Celebration in Central Florida. These visionaries did not neglect the health care needs of the community. They collaborated with the Florida Hospital Health System, part of the Adventist Health System, and Celebration Health was conceived. Florida Hospital Health System was a logical choice for several reasons: It has over 90 years of medical leadership serving Central Florida; it is Central Florida's largest health care provider; it is the largest integrated health system in the nation; and it is part of the Adventist Health System, a unique system founded on healthy lifestyle principles. These healthy lifestyle principles have been examined in a study of 50,000 people who have lived the lifestyle advocated by the Adventist Health System for 25 years. They were found to be among the healthiest people in the world.[15]

The Florida Hospital Health System was asked to address the needs of the community in creative and interactive ways and the Celebration Health facility became the anchor of the innovation in health and healing services. It is a unique setting that delivers hospital care, but its primary focus is on community care, wellness and disease prevention. The facility provides a location for physician offices and includes a major fitness center, rehabilitation center, community pharmacy and food service. In addition, it houses patient education and risk management programs that go beyond the usual reduction of risk behaviors and encompasses elements of life and health that create not only disease reduction or health promotion, but also optimum health. In its approach to treating the whole person, Celebration Health has incorporated eight guiding principles for individuals who are seeking a healthy life: Choice, Rest, Environment, Activities, Trust in God, Interpersonal

Relationships, Outlook and Nutrition.[16]

Patients, known as "guests," play a central, directive and interactive role in their care and health improvement plans. It is a mix of conventional customs and futuristic concepts where old-fashioned, individualized, personal attention is combined with the power of new technology and paradigms for caring. The setting is Disney-like in its quality, thoughtful planning and characterization as a center for creating and maintaining healthy lifestyles. The Celebration Health experience is consistent with the anticipated future of health care and certainly the direction in which today's empowered patient is moving. This model emphasizes holistic health and healing, and the health system provides individuals with facilities, staff and opportunities to experience optimum health at whatever their age and health status. The goal is for all people in the community, not only those who are ill and are the inpatient "guests," to achieve the best possible health outcomes from their encounters with healers.

The centerpiece of Celebration Health is a change from traditional models of care based on acute encounters with medicine to a focus on a healthy lifestyle integrated with the traditional health care competencies of primary, acute, surgical and emergency care. In this transition, Celebration Health recognizes the challenges facing health care today in which most health problems stem from diseases individuals bring on themselves from lifestyle choices and personal mismanagement of chronic conditions. The hallmark of Celebration Health care, however, is the recognition of the mutuality of the relationships between each of the players—the patient, the hospital and the community. In this shift, although the hospital may be the anchor for healing within the community, it is not the center of the care. It is but one player in a continuum of healing services that helps individuals change the way they live in order to successfully prevent and manage disease. Every component of the design and management of Celebration Health promotes this paradigm shift in the creation of healing for the community.

Engaging Other Healers in the Community Covenant

To promote the transformation of American health care, Celebration Health's leadership enlisted the support and collaboration of approximately 35 partners, all of whom are working cooperatively to integrate innovations in healing that support the goals of the community. These partnerships support Celebration

---

Health with a wide range of activities, programs and equipment to promote health. In return, these companies use this community setting to further develop and test the latest in technology, information services and patient support strategies. As a result, new methods are developed and then the center is used for training and demonstrations to other parts of the country.

Through the work of one of the partners, the Center for Health Futures, Celebration Health is a party to identifying, developing and assessing the effectiveness of new models of care. Wyeth-Ayerst works with Celebration Health to develop and maintain a Center for Women's Health Services. Women who receive obstetric and gynecologic services at physicians' offices on site have access to extensive web-based information services and are encouraged to research their questions and conditions prior to physician visits. Glaxo Wellcome works with Celebration Health to pioneer innovative disease management programs and outcomes research. One disease management initiative is a pilot program to better manage chronic headaches. This program identifies chronic headache sufferers, educates them to better understand their symptoms and the mechanisms that trigger pain and telephones them later to assess the success of the education in controlling their chronic headaches.

Glaxo Wellcome also worked with Celebration Health on a smoking cessation project. Celebration Health staff noticed that when patients were in the hospital, surrounded by concerned family, they were more receptive to education about smoking and quitting than at other times. This led to inpatient counseling for patient and family coupled with pharmaceutical care and resulted in quit rates twice those of other model programs. The AGFA Medical Division of Bayer developed the radiology department to meet the health care demands of the future and showcase a state-of-the-art Picture Archival Communications System (PACS) that creates the highest quality diagnostic images and simultaneously streamlines the diagnostic process. Celebration Health serves as a demonstration center for training other radiology departments now making the transition to digital technology. Ethicon Endo-Surgery, Inc., a Johnson & Johnson Company, showcases its surgical tools in the operating room, and uses it as a test site for new minimally invasive tools and services to advance surgical outcomes. Celebration Health will oversee educational programs on the Ethicon Endo-Surgery Mammotome Breast Biopsy System, demonstrated to be three times more accurate than a core needle biopsy. General

Electric Medical Systems was involved in early strategic discussions about Celebration Health's design and now is a center for GE Medical's state-of-the-art diagnostic imaging equipment. Approximately a dozen types of GE Medical's diagnostic imaging equipment can be found at Celebration Health, including the Stenoscope mobile digital imaging systems, the AMX-4+ mobile X-ray system, the Millennium MG multigeometry nuclear imaging system, the Advantx DRS integrated digital radiology system and the Signa Conquest MR system.

Reaching Out to the Surrounding Community

These Celebration Health project partners are impressive, the facility is beautiful, well equipped and well staffed. It is a center for health that reaches out to the central Florida area and to the nation—and eventually to the world. An example is a project with AstraZeneca, which partnered with Celebration Health to develop a Digestive Health Center in central Florida. The center is developing comprehensive best practice models in the care management of patients with gastrointestinal (GI) disorders, including outreach to the community to identify and treat patients with GI disease. This model will be replicated throughout the Florida Hospital Health System and Adventist Health System.

Another example of reaching out, this time to the Florida Governor's Office, was the formation of the Community Health Improvement Council (CHIC). The CHIC provides a committed infrastructure for addressing health and disease issues within the state and will invest $8 million over eight years into central Florida health improvements. As a result of working with the Governor's Office, new resources for health care, most recently for congestive heart failure, have received support in the state's budget. Since the CHIC membership also includes the Central Florida Health Care Coalition, a group composed of over 200 employers in the region and involving the largest employers in the nation, projects with employers are being planned.

Celebration Health has its critics. They argue that the facility and its service components are only possible because of the extensive partnerships with Disney and other corporations drawn to Orlando because of its tourist potential and Disney association. As a matter of fact, those elements have facilitated some of the interactions. The Orlando site is a preferred location for medical conventions, and Celebration Health can easily originate satellite-beamed surgeries and educational sessions into the Orlando Convention

Center where large numbers of clinicians are meeting. But in truth, it is the attitude of the leadership, not the location of the building, that makes Celebration Health what it is. It is the nature of the healer-patient and healer-community relationships that create the "green-field" for the experimentation and success that the organization clearly appears to be enjoying. Furthermore, no one at Celebration Health will claim that their relationships are truly unique, as they have learned in their work with other communities.

Reaching Out to Other Communities

Celebration Health and a number of other communities are charter members of the Accelerating Community Transformation— or ACT—Project.[17] ACT is a multidimensional, five-year applied research project guided by the broad and ambitious vision of building healthier communities, first in the United States and, ultimately, throughout the world. ACT builds community partnerships and civic infrastructures to achieve and demonstrate measurable improvements in community health and quality of life. The ACT Project has ambitious goals:

- To establish and refine community visions of healthy and sustainable futures;

- To develop clear statements of desired outcomes and how to achieve them;

- To develop a software tool to measure outcomes of community health in a standardized and efficient way and to link outcomes to performance;

- To measure and track indicators of community improvement; and

- To identify, create and document collaborative approaches and interventions "that work," creating a repertoire of "best practices" to increase health and quality of life that can be shared with other communities.

To date there are nearly thirty operative ACT sites in various stages of implementation in seventeen states. By design, the locations, social and economic characteristics and demographics of the ACT Project site communities are diverse and represent a cross section of America. They have a track record in applying the principles and values of healthier communities, and they want to further build capacity to improve health and quality of life. For example, two of the program sites illustrate the vast difference between the sites in the area of geography. One is a small, old, southern town with a population of approximately 25,000 that began as a health resort many years ago. All of the organizations and agencies involved in this project are located in a small vicinity; they are all familiar with one another, have established contacts and have worked together for many years. In contrast, another ACT site covers an area of approximately 10,000 square miles over 15 counties in 4 states.

In the course of their work, ACT communities are addressing pressing public and community health issues. One community ranked 50th in the United States in its rate of infant mortality when it began its healthy community initiative. Another community had lost 40% of its population in years immediately prior to the implementation of ACT due to unemployment when major employers pulled out of the area. In their projects, various communities are addressing low immunization rates among vulnerable populations; substance abuse; domestic and community violence; identification of and treatment for diseases such as asthma, cardiovascular conditions, diabetes and depression; and achieving Healthy People 2000 Objectives. The community goals, however, are not all health related, as other factors clearly influence health status. Some communities are focusing on improving regional economic health; increasing high school completion and GED attainment; developing workforces, job retraining, and adapting to changes in community jobs; decreasing homelessness and increasing affordable housing; improving racial and ethnic harmony; developing urban and community neighborhoods; improving cooperation and collaboration among community agencies; and improving transitions from school to work.

Like the other projects that represent emerging covenants, this one is new, but there are notable examples of progress in the ACT communities. The sense of leadership on the part of healers and reciprocity and responsibility on the part of communities defy the current wisdom about what change is possible in this country today. One community trained over 150 volunteers who are currently providing respite care to caregivers throughout the community. In another community, the ACT program instituted "community forums" to convene representatives from five or six towns in a single county to identify and collaborate on problem issues. In one of these forums, between 30% and 40% of the participants are high school teenagers. Student participation has given them a sense of their own leadership ability and provided the impetus to take responsibility for and ownership of their community.

ACT Community Outcomes Toolkit

The Outcomes Toolkit is a new software-supported methodology to design, organize and monitor measurable indicators of community health and quality of life.[18] It is a performance-based planning tool that incorporates the many stages of community development through a fully integrated software package. The Toolkit provides step-by-step guidance to its users to: create a shared vision, develop action plans, identify and define outcomes and indicators, set measurable targets, identify data sources and data collection methodologies, analyze results and generate reports. The Outcomes Toolkit grew from questions regarding what factors in a community affect the quality of life and health of individuals and which of those factors are amenable to change. Because of the pioneering nature of the Toolkit, its development involved qualitative research by a team of professionals who visited multiple ACT sites. The team included a cultural anthropologist, an ethnographer, public health and community development experts and others. The development process involved iterative steps in which the team designed, built and tested the software.

It fosters collaboration between public and private sectors and organizations and agencies by linking the continuum of community development activities through common goals, objectives, standards and data collection methods. The software is installed on multiple computers in organizations throughout a community to enhance data collection, organization and information sharing. The various sites using the Toolkit in a community are networked via the Internet to enable information sharing, data entry from multiple locations, the creation of outcome measures and a database incorporating data from the multiple sites. Participating ACT program organizations can use predefined outcome measures and/or establish their own indicators and, in doing so, use data from any number of primary or secondary sources. For example, a community might incorporate data from the health department, hospital and coroner's office in their community and compare it to national standards to measure and assess infant mortality rates.

The Outcomes Toolkit is an important project emerging from the partnership between Celebration Health and the Center for Health Futures because it allows for outreach to so many other communities throughout the nation, and perhaps eventually, throughout the world. It not only measures the traditional inputs,

processes and outcomes that support health care, but also addresses the measurement of outcomes related to education, criminal justice and the local economy, each of which are factors that contribute to the health of individuals and the community. In contrast
to patient level outcome measures, the use of outcome measurement at the community level is much less advanced, yet, increasingly, that is where health care decisions are being made. Thus,
the development and implementation of the Outcomes Toolkit is a
tangible contribution to measurement of outcomes in community
health, well being and quality of life in a standardized way. This
has been recognized by a number of organizations who are now
in the process of exploring the use of the Outcomes Toolkit, including the Centers for Disease Control, United Way, local Chambers
of Commerce and a number of community foundations.

Covenant and the Pressing Needs of the Future

Every one of the examples mentioned here—whether individuals,
organizations, companies or communities—takes a step in the
direction of covenants and, in most cases, covenants of obligation
with the partners they engage for the benefit of healing. Every one
of the examples could be criticized for not taking enough steps into
the fullness of an explicit covenant, but to do so would be coun-
terproductive to fully exploring covenants and caring today. The
success of these covenants should be celebrated and the new challenges ahead examined. It is more important to find the ways to
support them, as the needs for the future are so great.

As we confront the growth of consumer-driven and empowered health care demands, the growing number of therapeutic
alternatives arising from research, the pace of faster e-commerce
lifestyles and the aging of the population, the models of care we
have traditionally known will be less viable. The foundations of the
values and the ethics will not, however. As noted elsewhere, what
is gained in information has been lost in wisdom. It is in the wisdom of the covenant healer that we may well find the answers to
the complexity we fear will overwhelm us in this new millennium.
These healers and the relationships they are crafting with patients
and communities are well worth preserving, enabling and modeling.

Chapter 9

Healing Health Care

Crafting Covenants in the New Millennium

> *Health policies are rarely derived from explicit and systematic analysis of the moral values that shape them. Much of the art of national and international politics consists in structuring decision-making in such a way that value issues are not confronted. The aim is to keep peace between, and within, divergent belief systems. However, once framed, a health policy unerringly reveals the values that drive a society; and these cannot escape examination retrospectively.*[1]

Edmund Pellegrino

Coming Full Circle

This book ends where it began, back in Greece in 1984, where ethicists and academics, government representatives from many nations, theologians from the world's religions and experts from the clinical and scientific disciplines of medicine and public health engaged in a dialogue about health policy and human values. The group explored how ethical and religious values affected the health policy decisions of the world's nations. Dr. Pellegrino was one of the medical ethicists whose observations shaped the discussions. It was at that meeting that he made the comment quoted above. His reflection was true to the exploration of national health policy at that time, and it remains true in health care practices and national health care policy today. The policies that have shaped the nation's care over the important and fast-moving decades of the last half-century did not explicitly address the covenant relationships among those who were a party to them—or should have been. As a nation and within our clinical relationships, we did not confront the values that framed the foundation of the healer-patient relationship. We did not examine the responsibilities of patients and communities towards themselves and each other for the quality of their own health and healing. Yet, it is possible, now, to look back and retrospectively assess what happened to the covenants that were the basis for the health and aspects of personal and community life. It is possible to determine how and when the covenant in health care was lost and how policies and practices might have been enriched if covenants had been engaged.

Had we engaged in covenant-building, we might not have left so many of our dying in intractable pain and hounded so many of our healers for treating them. We might not have neglected the perspectives of the animal rights activists so long that some would resort to extreme positions and strategies, threatening researchers, and leaving potentially solvable disease problems suspended in damaged labs and destroyed data. Had we felt the reciprocity in the healer patient relationship, we might never have transformed our insurance systems into no-fault financing systems, removing much of the incentives for patient self-care and prevention. Had we acknowledged the obligations of communities, we would not have allowed our public health infrastructure to crumble or become so eager to assume that healers, captive to capitation payment systems, would absorb the increasing costs associated with social problems. If we recognized the importance of the covenantal trust between patient and healer, we might not sell and resell encounter data without the knowledge of either, or for a purpose to which neither had explicitly agreed. If we and others were globally in an international covenant of caring, we might have approached the problems in pharmaceutical donations differently—not as a rationale for pummeling the donors, but as an opportunity to save lives and improve health systems.

If covenants of obligation become more explicit in our relationships, we might more satisfactorily resolve the problems we face in health care today:

- If traditional healers—allopathic physicians—felt more "in covenant" with other healers, would they be more willing to embrace nontraditional healers and methods and bring them into their practices? Would they be more accepting of direct-to-consumer advertising as an educational and compliance strategy with an appropriate place in health care? Would they be more open to nurse practitioners and other nonphysicians who provide care to the uninsured who lack access to care?

- If alternative healers felt more "in covenant" with patients, would they limit the claims associated with their practices to those truly demonstrated as valid, avoiding the potentially ineffective and potentially harmful approaches that may be philosophically attractive, but not genuinely beneficial to health?

- If the news media felt more "in covenant" with patients and communities, would they improve the quality of reporting and develop methods to assure accuracy in reporting on the health care arena?

- If communities felt more "in covenant," would they comprehensively address the social problems of racial, ethnic and gender bias that drives violence and higher utilization of health care? Would they protect the young and the old with safer streets? Would they work towards cleaner air and living conditions to prevent asthma disability?

- If citizens of the nation felt "in covenant" with each other and our healers, would we be more inclined to contribute to tax-supported or other pools to insure those who cannot afford care? Would we be more willing to adhere to lifestyle and health care practices that control costs? Would we be willing to require that each of us do so? Would we require that, much like children who receive immunizations for school entry, the elderly be likewise immunized against preventable adult diseases to be eligible for Medicare coverage?

- If patients and communities felt "in covenant" with our healers, would they be more willing to see their own role in shaping the status of their health and the shape of their wallets? Would we recognize that our own behaviors and the health of the communities we live in also play a role in the quality of our lives, the status of our health and the cost of our care?

Whatever the problems in the headlines today, in the years to come the challenges for health care will become greater. The public may focus on the immediate concerns of cost, quality and access to care, but those in the healing enterprises know that there are a number of fundamental questions that have only begun to emerge:

- How will we support the academic health centers that train new healers and research disease without full funding of biomedical research projects or the patient care dollars to support the effort?

- How will bioethical and biogenetic decisions be made as the science and technology of health care outstrips the capacity of this nation to address its values and craft legislation accordingly?

- How will the healing and health care financing needs of an aging baby-boomer society be met?

- To what degree will alternative therapies be legitimized, not through research but due to patient demand and willingness to self-pay? Will the impact of these therapies be positive on healing, health care costs and mainstream clinical care?

- What is the likelihood that the nation will be confronted with emerging infections, increasing antibiotic resistance and bio-terrorism? To what degree will those factors change the safety of cities and threaten the public's health?

- How will the growing number of clinical and pharmaceutical solutions to lifestyle desires, choices and problems be financed?

- How will those sectors outside health care, particularly those in the financial and electronic commerce industries, affect the course of healing?

Only One Step along the Way

The meeting in Athens was the beginning of this exploration into the roots of healing within cultures and the importance of covenants in healing relationships. This last chapter will not be the end of either; it is merely a stop along the way. It is my intention that this review of our collective healing history will result in a dialogue about covenants, and that new covenants will emerge in today's healing enterprises—thus, shaping our healing future. It appears to me that there are principles in ancient covenants relevant to health care today that will help us craft a covenant-centered future.

Principle Number One: Covenants Flow from the Senior Party and Are Preceded by Gifts

Before inviting someone into a covenant, gifts are given. We in this country cannot deny that we are among the most gifted and privileged of all the people in the world. We enjoy the freedom that democracy assures. Our healing enterprise grew from that democracy, the resources have been plentiful and gifts have flowed abundantly. The nation has developed extraordinary scientific and healing resources and possesses the talent and the technology to shape a better health future for all people—not just for the "insured" patients or for those living in our country, but also for people lacking the resources for care here and overseas. It has crafted the sciences and the systems that make a difference in our own lives and the lives of others. For all the complaints about the state of health care today, we should not ignore the reality of the gifts we have received from our healers and should acknowledge that we have asked for and have received the most well-endowed health care system on the globe. For all the problems in health services, there remain more opportunities than there are obstacles. Our healers have given gifts to us as individual patients, as well. They have studied hard, worked long hours, taken personal risks, contributed their talents and produced many of the miracles that were asked of them. These gifts, given and received, form the basis of the early covenants that were established here and that should evolve into the basis of new covenants of obligation. It was healers, through their oaths, who invited us into covenants and, by virtue of their expertise, remain the senior parties today. It is the healers who should now take the lead in proposing the new covenant. There are some who may believe that healers are no longer the senior parties or, by virtue of the current patient-empowered climate, should not retain the rights of such expert positioning within the proposal of covenants. For all the faults of healing in health care today, however, our healers remain the most skilled of all the parties at living within the covenants of the oaths they have taken. Unlike the rest of us, they understand covenants in a way that patients and communities do not. They are, therefore, the best teachers and leaders into a covenant lifestyle that the future demands.

Principle Number Two: Covenants Do Not End

If covenants are embraced, neither this nor any other effort to explore them can be the end of the story. The beginning of a covenant can be dated; the ending cannot. Covenants are established and they evolve. They should not wither. They do not die. There is no "stepping outside" of the covenant for a vacation or a "break." Covenants, established by our forbears in healing, have framed relationships between healers and patients for generations. Healers passed down their healing ethic to subsequent generations of healers, sharing even the specific oaths to serve patients. As oaths are revitalized today, healers are signaling to the patients and communities that the covenant created thousands of years ago is still the basis of the healing relationships by which healers themselves wish to live. There are no exit clauses in covenants. There are no buy-out provisions in covenants. To paraphrase Professor May, once a person abides in a covenant, he does not step outside it. Do it well or do it poorly, do it awake or do it in sleep, the covenant role endures. Just as healers practice their skills and are available to patients at all times, so, too, should patients and communities practice their roles continually. Healthy behaviors are no less a concern when buying groceries, driving a car or watching television than they are during office visits to the physician. Once engaged in a covenant of obligation, healing will be "top-of-mind" for patients and communities, not just for the healers who serve them.

Principle Number Three: Covenants Change Over Time

At the beginning of a covenant, it is impossible to know where the relationship will lead and what the covenant relationship will require of its parties. It is this element of evolution that distinguishes covenants from contracts. Contracts spell out every step and, even at the beginning, define the end. Covenants, by definition, cannot do this. It is impossible to say how each party will influence the other and how the needs and demands upon those involved will change. In the present, many of the parties to healing are re-examining the nature of the healing enterprise and the relationships involved. It would be wise for all concerned that this examination results in new covenant of obligation relationships among the many healers in health care today, between healers and patients, and between healers and communities. When newly-defined healers accept their responsibilities to the covenant, they will be more likely to shape positive health care climates. If patients and communities accept responsibilities and obligations, they will help carry the load that has been shouldered so predominately by healers. The relationships that create healing and quality health care outcomes will become the shared responsibility of everyone. Currently, some of the players central to the healing enterprises are able to ignore their roles as healers. In the future, having accepted a covenant of obligation, none of the parties will be able to shift their responsibilities to others and expect that healing will simply be "granted."

Coming into Covenants of Obligation

Covenants of obligation address the challenges of the new millennium. The existing covenants of grant should be replaced with the more mature covenants of obligation. We as a nation are not satisfied with the health care services we receive. We want more and better care. We demand new advances in research, and we are

---

worried about how we will pay for it. The old covenants of grant that existed between healers and patients have run their course and are no longer sufficient for our health care challenges. The old covenants of grant did not effectively engage all those involved in healing. They did not engage the patients and the communities that are such an important determinant of health today. In order to satisfy the nation's wants, we must acknowledge that all those who "practice" within the healing enterprise—healers, patients and communities—achieve health and healing within mutually supportive relationships.

Each party must feel obligated to the other. Each party to the covenant must be willing to reciprocate with the other in the healing process. Each must be willing to do his part in finding the best solution to the important lifestyle, policy, political and business decisions that are pending at the beginning of the new millennium. These solutions will shape the future of our health and that of other nations, as well. None of us—healer, patient or community—can expect that health care will be healed unless we all participate. None of us can expect to be insulated from the consequences of our behavior. Whether we are patients, healers or communities, we cannot shun the opportunity that a covenant of obligation in healing can create. Mutual obligations will benefit us all.

If covenants, particularly covenants of obligation, are to be the order of the future, how will this be accomplished? Who will be party to these covenants? What processes and documents will frame them? How will those who wish to engage in covenants prepare for them and execute them? Will everyone embrace covenants? Can they be required to do so? What about those who may reject the invitation to join in covenant and what are our responsibilities to them?

Creating covenants of obligation will require six essential conditions. Some of these are obvious and will be familiar to those who have developed new programs and projects. Some are well-honed skills of healers, patient advocates and community leaders. These skills draw upon the leadership development, strategic planning, policy making and other processes already used by those in the health care community.

First, there must be an *intention* to develop and enter into a covenant of obligation. Being in a covenant is no accident. It will not occur because one "just happens" to be in a particular job or position in the health care arena, because one has made an appointment to visit a healer, or because one is a resident of a community. Compare it to a wedding and a marriage. A marriage does not "happen" because a man and a woman show up in church at the appointed hour. The marriage covenant is struck because both parties have committed to going forward in their relationship over time. Particularly on the part of the party who first proposes the marriage, or covenant, the intention must be clear—it must be intentional. As the expert party who makes the proposal, healers must have the intention to form covenants with each other, with their patients and with communities. Without that intention, the next steps cannot and will not be taken.

The second essential condition calls for *a purging of the immediate past,* a clearance, or "letting go" of any biases that might interfere with new styles of relating. This includes releasing the prejudges, ideas, likes and dislikes about the past relationships. Emptying out will free the mind and the heart to consider new ways of relating to the covenant in general and relating to the parties who will become part of the covenant specifically. This will not be easy. Large numbers of interlocking contracts are in place. These contracts are layered over old, dysfunctional covenants of grant. Biases between patients, healers and communities are strong and many of them are negative. It will not be possible to engage in covenants if we continue to believe that patients are irresponsible and ignorant, healers are greedy and unethical and communities are disengaged and disinterested. New covenants require new ideas and a past that is purged, resolved and left behind. New covenants require a fresh start and a clean slate.

A third essential condition prescribes that covenants must be *rooted.* The best roots for grasping covenants of obligation are those from the ancient past. Today's health care ground is, frankly, not sacred enough for a covenant of obligation to be proposed, root and grow again. Our ground has been eroded and is no longer fertile soil in which to plant a practice as paradigm-shifting and potentially radical as a covenant of obligation. As the modern scientific era and the wealth of the nation produced its fruits, the old covenants of grant could have matured into covenants of obligation. They did not. Instead, the existing covenants of grant began to break down, burdened by new, complex and interlocking contractual arrangements that characterized changes in health financing over the past 50 years, for instance. New players in health care, policy, politics, insurance, advertising, media and electronic communications did not recognize themselves as healers, did not embrace the healer's covenant, or adopt healing roles.

Patients and communities did not mature into accepting responsibilities for the state of their own health. The confluence of these factors in this modern era limits our ability to mature our healing covenants towards those of obligation to one another. Perhaps by returning to the sacredness of healing and the interdependence of the relationships, the roots of healing can take hold again in fertile soil.

New covenants must be *connected* for the fourth essential condition. Interconnections with those in the covenant of obligation are essential to maintaining it. Hippocrates was wise in holding physicians accountable to one another in a covenant of obligation. Those relationships of obligation supported the difficult demands of research, learning and practice. The obligation to one another assured that no physician was left without peers in the demanding arenas of science and skill that were called for in healing. This should stand as a lesson for those developing and engaging in covenants of obligation today, whether patients, healers or communities. Maintaining and restoring health, and treating and healing disease cannot be accomplished without the connections to other patients, healers and communities. Each party to the covenant will perform better within a covenant and will meet his obligations more completely if he reciprocates with others in peer relationships. Much as healers gain support for the demands of their roles by connecting with other healers, so, too, will patients gain support by connecting with other patients and communities. Each party will do well within covenants if he contributes something to the healing of others, for it is frequently in giving that we receive the most.

The fifth essential condition demands that those who develop and work within covenants must *pause* from time to time to reconsider the relationship. The work of health care is demanding, and recreating covenants will make the tasks of healing even more so. The call for covenants is intended to ease the crises we will most certainly face without them, but covenants are hard work. They require near constant attention to the ebbs and flows of human relations. Covenants are not intellectual constructs, but heart-focused, soul-driven lifestyles. Covenants are not only for the good of the patient, but for the good of the healer as well. Overworked, stressed-out, and unhealthy healers cannot give what they do not have. Patients whose lives have been altered by disease or who face critical care crises need the pause to sort out what changes they want and are willing to seek from their healers. Communities, too, will change as economic circumstances, employment, immigration and disasters take hold. Covenants are destined to change. It is, therefore, important that from time to time the parties to the covenants reconsider and recommit to them. This takes an occasional pause to reassess their workings to determine if changes are needed. Some couples do this within marriage. They reassess their relationship to determine if changes should be made. Not a bad idea for covenants in health care, as well.

The sixth and final essential condition asks that covenants cause the parties to *stretch* into and beyond their capabilities in creating, sustaining and healing their health and the health of others. If we are to embrace an idea as fundamental and radical as covenant, we should set our sights high. We should call out the best in ourselves as patients, healers and communities. We should seek the best within the relationships we have. Too often in health care we have limited the capacity to do better, believing that we cannot, or that others around us cannot, successfully perform to the goal. Yet, the history of health care is one of remarkable progress on all fronts. New funds have appeared from private, public and commercial sources to build the infrastructures wanted, healers have adapted their practices to what the nation wanted, and new medicines have spilled out of pipelines with increasing regularity. Today, there is tremendous wealth and diversity in personnel and resources. The health workforce is one of the overall, best educated groups of all the sectors of the economy. It is already bound by covenant. These resources are not some albatross around the neck of the nation, but the wings that soar to new heights of healing. Covenant may well be one of the flight paths towards the change we so desire today.

Who Should Create New Covenants of Obligation?

Donald Berwick, of the Institute for Health Care Improvement, says that all those who "shape the experience of patients and the social investment in care" should be party to the ethical ideals of healers.[2] I agree. Even though he is referring to "ethics" and I to "covenant," our perspectives are so similar as to be indistinguishable. I'll be more specific. Everyone who works in a professional or volunteer position in a healing enterprise should define him- or herself as a healer, should be a party to a covenant and should adopt a covenant of obligation in relation to the patients they serve. This is independent of the education or position of those healers. It is independent of whether the healer serves one patient or a million patients. It is independent of whether the service is clerical or clinical. It is independent of whether the patient served is a single individual or the collective whole. As a result, I include physicians and policy makers, surgeons and clerks,[3] legislators and litigators, advertisers and e-commerce entrepreneurs. I also include newscasters, insurance company clerks and pharmaceutical sales representatives. These individuals form the initial covenants of obligation—those that exist among healers and are at the foundation of all the other covenants. These are the senior parties. They are the framers of the covenants of obligation. They will invite each other and others—the patients and the communities—into the reciprocal relationships that will create the covenant of obligation called for.

The creation of these covenants will not happen by myth or by magic. The identity as a healer, the intention to create covenants and act within them will not assure that they arise full-grown like some goddess of old from the head of her father. The creation of these new covenants of obligation will emerge from a new generation of leaders in health care who may now be appearing on the scene. These are leaders worthy of being nurtured by the rest of us. These are leaders whose intentions will span beyond the limits of the sitting President and congressional majority. They are not leaders who will deliver solutions, but the leaders who will facilitate the processes to find solutions. They will be able, at all times, to see the viewpoint of others, to believe in the value of collaboration and synergy, to resolve conflicts and to park their egos at the door. They will articulate the necessity of making sacrifices for the good of the whole nation, for those served and for those who serve. Health care today is on the verge of change from external forces, particularly from the information technology and e-commerce sectors. The leadership required to manage the challenges will come from the most covenant-centered individuals if it emerges from inside of health care. This leadership will have communication and peace-building skills that will enable us to come together long enough to work past the cynicism in our attitudes today. These leaders will be, in their core, healers. They will understand that healing, especially healing a chronically ill patient like today's health care system, does not happen overnight, that they must be cautious and, most of all, do no further harm.

These leaders will, first of all, heal health care. They will help create the sanctuaries of tolerance for bringing today's healers together to search for their commitment to covenant. Once they are united in trust, they will use that emotional glue to approach patients and communities. Since patients carry with them the vestiges of the covenants established throughout history, they will be inclined to welcome the invitation to participate.

What Will a Covenant of Obligation Look Like?

A covenant of obligation will be an explicit statement of relationship. It will be reciprocal. I have only been able to locate one healer with a clear statement of such a covenant. The staff and patients of Indiana Health Centers, Inc. developed it.[4] This healer is a community health center composed of clinical sites and satellites. It is a safety-net provider established to care for the uninsured, the underinsured and those lacking access to care. As a Community Health Center (CHC), it is dedicated to serving those too often at the margins of our communities. If healers can create covenants of obligation within these settings and amidst the resource constraints of caring for the poor and the disadvantaged, we all can.

Their covenant of obligation addresses access, affordability, quality, convenience, prevention and dignity. It says:

Each Indiana Health Centers person promises...	Your responsibility is...
...to provide quality to keep you healthy	...to schedule and keep your services appointments for immunizations, annual exams, WIC and cancer and other screenings
...to provide quality nutrition and WIC services, as well as quality medical care when you are ill, and to have a medical provider you can reach by telephone when we are closed	...to call us when you have a health problem or nutritional concern
...to be open at times that work for you, including evenings and weekends	...to let us know if our evening and weekend hours work for you
...to make every attempt to honor appointment times	...to make appointments whenever possible, to make appointments at convenient time, to make every effort to be on time for an appointment, and to call if you can't keep your appointment

...to take a personal interest in your health and keep all personal information private	...to give us accurate information about you and your health, and to make sure we can always contact you if necessary
...to treat you with respect and courtesy	...to treat us and other clients with respect and courtesy
...to ask for and consider your input	...to complete the client satisfaction survey
...to keep the cost as low as possible	...to pay your fees for medical services when due, to tell us if you have any insurance coverage, to take advantage of any health insurance program you might qualify for, to provide us with accurate financial information
...to refer you to other services that would be helpful	...to consider using the referral and let us know if it works for you
...to offer many services that help you stay well	...to use as many of our services at each visit as possible

Other covenants may be stated in different terms because they will be uniquely structured to fit the nature of those within the relationship. The covenant of caring that emergency personnel have with their communities will differ from those that primary care physicians have with patients and families. The covenant that health care trade association staffs have with their members will differ from those that their members have with the patients and communities they serve. The covenant of state public health officials will be different in times of crises than in times of quiescence.

Some covenants may be totally personal—as between a healer and a patient. Some may be organizational—as between a hospital and a community. Since oaths have been used to structure and define covenants, most parties will choose to state their covenants in that way. Covenants won't be the answer to every dilemma, but it will be the starting point for resolving many. These covenants will probably be short, so that they are easily remembered. It is not the document, after all, that will be important, but the degree to which the reciprocal promises live in the hearts and inform the heads of those who are party to it. These covenants will

also provide for some sort of reconciliation process, as everyone is fallible and will fail to live up to the spirit of the covenant on occasion. Building back the trust and re-entering the relationship will require the parties to restore their standing in the covenant when it breaks down.

Covenants in Action

Do covenants work? Do they make a difference in practice? For true covenants of obligation, it is not yet clear. So few can be identified and none are so longstanding that they can be measured at this point. Many hospitals and health care institutions now post patient rights and, less often, patient responsibility statements, but only the Indiana Health Centers, Inc. stands as a true, reciprocal covenant of obligation developed between healers and patients. In addition to the covenant of grant established in the Hippocratic Oath, which has been measured and found to have a positive impact on practice,[5] there are three others worthy of note and discussion. One is from a corporation, one is from an association and the other is from an individual.

The first is the Johnson & Johnson Credo. This credo is typical of a covenant of grant, but it is notable because its impact has been measured.[6] It reads:

Our Credo

We believe our first responsibility is to the doctors, nurses and patients, to mothers and all others who use our products and services. In meeting their needs everything we do must be of high quality. We must constantly strive to reduce our costs in order to maintain reasonable prices. Customers' orders must be serviced promptly and accurately. Our suppliers and distributors must have an opportunity to make a fair profit.

We are responsible to our employees, the men and women who work with us throughout the world. Everyone must be considered as an individual. We must respect their dignity and recognize their merit. They must have a sense of security in their jobs. Compensation must be fair and adequate, and working conditions clean, orderly and safe. Employees must feel free to make suggestions and complaints. There must be equal opportunity for employment, development, and advancement for those qualified. We must provide competent management, and their actions must be just and ethical.

We are responsible to the communities in which we live and

work and to the world community as well. We must be good citizens—support good works and charities and bear our fair share of taxes. We must encourage civic improvements and better health and education. We must maintain in good order the property we are privileged to use, protecting the environment and natural resources.

Our final responsibility is to our stockholders. Business must make a sound profit. We must experiment with new ideas. Research must be carried on, innovative programs developed and mistakes paid for. New equipment must be purchased, new facilities provided and new products launched. Reserves must be created to provide for adverse times. When we operate according to these principals, the stockholder should realize a fair return.

In this credo, Johnson & Johnson, as a corporation, holds itself accountable to patients, family members, employees, communities and stockholders. It grants them quality products, working opportunities, good neighbor relations and returns on investment. It was written in the mid-1940s by the late Robert Wood Johnson, the company's leader, and was the guiding principal of his own management of the company. In 1972 it was the theme of the company's annual report and the basis of a series of meetings for company employees, led by the new chairman, Philip B. Hoffman. The credo formed a number of important corporate decisions, including the decision to maintain its headquarters in an urban area and support the redevelopment of the city rather than flee to more desirable settings in the country. The credo was tested most severely in 1982 when a criminal poisoning of Tylenol® resulted in a number of deaths. The company encountered a crisis of unprecedented proportions. No crisis management plan could have anticipated the turn of events and the demands on the company to cooperate with so many government officials, press contacts, consumers and customers. The company and a number of knowledgeable observers credit the credo with guiding corporate actions through the hour-by-hour responses that, within five months, led to its re-launch of Tylenol® into the marketplace, the repackaging of consumer goods to prevent similar tampering and the recapturing of 70% of the market it had previously held.

In another example, the National Health Council, an association of over 100 health groups, developed concepts of patient rights and responsibilities. The Council is composed of both patient and healer organizations and these rights and responsibilities were developed through extensive research with patients across the country. This statement, like the one developed by Indiana Health Centers, Inc., moves in the direction of reciprocity between healers and their patients.

All patients have the right to:

1. Informed consent in treatment decisions, timely access to specialty care, and confidentiality protections.

2. Concise and easily understood information about their coverage.

3. Know how coverage payment decisions are made and how they can be fairly and openly appealed.

4. Complete and easily understood information about the costs of their coverage and care.

5. A reasonable choice of providers and useful information about provider options.

6. Know what provider incentives or restrictions might influence practice patterns.

All patients, to the extent capable, have the responsibility to:

7. Pursue healthy lifestyles.

8. Become knowledgeable about their health plans.

9. Actively participate in decisions about their health care.

10. Cooperate fully on mutually accepted courses of treatment.[7]

In the final example, an individual, Martin Wasserman, M.D., J.D., at his swearing-in as Secretary of the Maryland Department of Health and Mental Hygiene, crafted a "Health Pledge to the People."

- To protect and promote the health of the public by creating healthy people in healthy communities

- To strengthen partnerships between the state and local government, the business community, and all of the health care providers in Maryland

- To build a world class and professional organization grounded in the principles of quality, accountability, cultural sensitivity, and efficiency.

This pledge, particularly the second item, established an explicit covenant of obligation among a broader group of healers and others within the state. The state's Department of Health and

Mental Hygiene reached out to form a relationship between community health departments, healers and communities through businesses. It was not only the guiding force of the state's department of health efforts, but 24 local health officers and 17 facilities also signed the pledge, and it was supported by over 200 quality teams. As a result, the Department of Health and Mental Hygiene was the only department-wide winner of the Governor's Gold Quality Award in 1997, which was based on the Baldridge quality award criteria. No other department in Maryland has won that award since. In addition, it formed the basis for extensive outreach to communities. When the Health Care Financing Administration approved a Medicaid waiver for the State of Maryland in record time, it commented that the state had secured the highest involvement of the public in any state up to that point. The state continues to involve the public, respecting citizen time by scheduling meetings in multiple locations so that no individual must travel more than one hour to participate.[8]

Evolution of Covenants Over Time

Those who engage each other in covenant terms are changed by the nature of their relationships. Much like young couples who marry with ideal expectations and later face difficult realities, each party to a covenant is challenged in ways that would not have been possible had they not entered into the covenant in the first place.

In healer-patient covenants in clinical settings neither party knows, at the outset, how the relationship will unfold. What diseases will befall the patient? What diagnostics or therapeutics will the healer be called upon to use? How rapidly will health care technology develop? How will the interaction between the two parties change each one as they work together over the years for the benefit of the patient's health—and perhaps for the healer's health as well? What will each party teach the other?

In a healer-community relationship neither party knows how the other will be required to change perspective in order to advance the covenant. How will communities respond to a healer's call for better education and social issue management to address, for example, problems of drug abuse, teen pregnancy, smoking and obesity driving health care costs? How will healers respond to the problems of violence that lead to increased health care utilization? How will the cost of caring for the uninsured be distributed among the community and its healers during economic recessions and high unemployment?

In the case of the patient-community relationship the evolution is even more uncertain. How will communities be defined? To which community does a patient belong? To the one in which they are employed, where they live or where they worship? To what degree are local employers a part of the community that should be engaged in solutions to health problems? Who will act as the voice of the community and have the "standing" to bring various groups within the community together to improve health? What are the limits of community control in the case where the community also feels responsibility for health care? Are there limits to the degree that a community and its healers should feel responsible for individual patients, including those who may not be inclined to practice healthy behaviors or respond within the covenant themselves?

No Easy Answers

By now, some readers are hoping for some final answers, and perhaps some easy answers, at that. However, this book was not intended as a scholarly analysis of the history of medicine, the ethics of medical care, or the theology of covenants. It was not intended to describe each of the health care issues of the day and present an analysis complete with prescriptive solutions. In fact, discussing such a scholarly analysis of even one of the dilemmas discussed here would require several volumes, as the field of health care publications readily demonstrates. This was intended to be a practical exploration of selected pivotal issues for healers, patients and communities interested in understanding and influencing the important decisions in the public policies of tomorrow's health care. This was intended to raise the questions that could frame discussions for those who are parties to the covenant that may be the better way to create the future. Each of the issues we face in health care today is a long-term work in progress. Each one is complex enough that none is likely to be resolved in the near future. Pausing now to consider how covenants may lead to solutions is the next important step along this path of healing health care. Pausing to develop covenants where they are most needed will be the best prescription for the maladies that ail our failing health care system. Covenants created by those in health care will help to resolve the conflicts that seem so intractable to us now.

This book was not intended to tinker at the margins of new health care financing proposals. There are very talented and dedicated people in the policy arena and health care enterprise who are crafting the incremental changes that will make health care accessible and affordable for decades to come. I cannot contribute to those efforts except by raising issues of covenant and suggesting that mutual obligations among all the players within health care will help. This book is instead, intended to radically challenge the nature of the relationships that are the foundations of health care today. On a new footing in relationships, the payment and financing issues can be more productively and easily addressed.

Furthermore, this book was not intended to tinker with the margins of health care companies. To do so would not help the future, it would harm it. Investors have long recognized that the health sector contributed to the economy in a number of ways. Health care has produced a growing number of jobs for an expanding workforce and kept the nation in the forefront of development as well. Health care was founded on solid science and increasingly productive, exportable technology. Demand-driven care has been good for health care. New technologies replaced old ones with greater effectiveness and, over time, efficiency. Health care contributed to more than national pride, but to a favorable balance of trade.

This book was not intended to shoot at a single, clear target with magic bullets. The targets in health care are too numerous, too fast moving, and there are no magic bullets. This book was not intended to offer specific solutions or to propose changes to "fix" health care—save one. It is my contention that if health care is to be healed, everyone involved in the healing enterprises of the day—the healers themselves, patients and communities—must enter into new and reinvigorated covenant relationships. Any reader who has made it through the entire text has encountered over three hundred questions in its various chapters. Yes, there have been precious few answers. But there are ways to reach towards those answers and find the right ones. The best way, I believe, is to reach back into the roots of healing and covenants— specifically covenants of obligation. What better time than at the start of the new millennium?

Epilogue
Questions about Covenants in Health Care

Writing this book has been an examination of the health care enterprise with its ancient roots from a new perspective. I enjoyed exploring the role that covenants can play in recreating the relationships necessary for healing ventures in the future. Along the way, I've had numerous discussions with others about this project. Most of the discussions were with healers, whether they were members of the audience at presentations on this topic or reviewers of drafts of this text. These individuals have been generous with their time and willingness to imagine health care with covenants of obligation as a core principle. Their willingness was not surprising to me, as so many healers already ascribe to an oath to guide their practices.

Some of the discussions have been with patients. Their reactions have been ultimately positive, as well, and that has surprised me. After venting their anger over the state of health care today, they readily accepted the notion that they, too, are responsible for their health, and that they have been less than faithful to the self-care and lifestyle choices that would improve their health and reduce the costs of care. Both groups—physicians and patients—were equally frustrated and looking for a solution. Both feel vulnerable. Neither wants health care wars to escalate.

All of these discussions challenged my thinking about covenants and this manuscript. Each discussion raised questions that are best addressed at the end, because they frame the future of a covenant-focused dialogue so well.

Why invite controversy by discussing the animal research debate?
I'll deal with the toughest question first. It was the most difficult to resolve and involved the most soul searching. One reviewer suggested removing the chapter on animal research, advising that the issue was contentious enough to create distractions that would interrupt the other messages on the central premises of the book.

It was a tough call to decide to keep that chapter. I have high regard for the views of this advisor. He is right: The issues involved in subjecting animals to research procedures for the benefit of humans (and other animals) may create controversy. However, I feel a responsibility to the health policy community, to researchers, to patients in need of research-driven cures, and even to my friends in the animal welfare community, to attempt to bring some peace to this issue by including their concerns in the context of covenant. To do less is to ignore my responsibility to each of them as a health policy analyst, observer and negotiator. I hope they will likewise feel a responsibility—I am inviting a covenant here—to engage in a discussion of the issues and not in the politics of personal destruction. I hope all the stakeholders involved will consider dealing with each other and their constituencies within a covenant that respects the views and obligations of each. I hope they will value my intention to assist with a resolution to this important arena of ethics, research and respect for all concerned. As in all the issues, it should be clear that there is much at stake.

Why address an international issue? Aren't our own issues compelling enough?
The reason I've chosen to deal with the problems of the developing world is to place our own problems, opportunities and assets in a broader perspective. I believe the chapter on drug donations is important because it so clearly calls for an evaluation of our values as human beings and as Americans, whose wealth relative to the rest of the world gives us the ability to help others. Helping others in such dire need allows us to reconnect with our humanity and the importance of compassion. In addition, helping those around the world sensitizes us to the needs of the poor at home.

Lending our assistance and donating our technologies to those abroad satisfies the needs I believe we all have to view healing as a gift to be shared, not a commodity to be bargained. It is also an inroad to creating global health, peace and prosperity. To help is not just good will, it is good health, good business, good policy and good politics.

Finally, I fear that health policy today is in danger of devolving into tactical elements of program operations, PMPMs[1], "cap" rates and budget requirements. The health care enterprise is much more complex, multifaceted, demanding and global than the current and most pressing concerns of today's budget battles. Unless we address these longer-term and more global issues today, the problems brewing outside our borders will become domestic

---

crises, and we will be unprepared to address them.

Why aren't there more prescriptions and specific directions?

By definition, only the parties to the covenant can work out the specifics. I've been about as specific as I can in the policy examples. I've suggested who the parties to the covenant might be and have pointed them in a direction. Only they can determine if they want to walk the path. Once underway, they'll decide how fast to progress and whether to detour from the route. Taking the first steps will not be easy, but the next steps will be even harder and no observer can second-guess the results.

It is along the way in the covenant relationship that the toughest questions must be addressed. These are the questions that we have avoided so well in the past several decades. These are questions of reciprocity and responsibility: If a patient can sue a managed care provider for failure to provide care (e.g., experimental therapies not covered by contract), can managed care sue patients for failure to follow medical advice? If employers cover the cost of a flu shot, can they deny sick leave to employees who chose not to be immunized but then get the flu? If the nation allows its citizens to carry guns, can insurers levy a surcharge for emergency room costs in areas of high gun ownership?

Talking about covenant is easy. Living covenant is not. As proof of that, I have been cautioned that my proposal for covenants is likely to be controversial enough as it is, even among physicians, who fare best in the analysis here. I did not begin to write with a bias toward any group, but over the course of my research and this examination, I became sympathetic to physicians and managed care. It strikes me that public policy has presented them an impossible task: provide, in some parental fashion, for all the desires of patients and communities who are insulated from the payment for care and the consequences of decisions. Nonetheless, I have been warned that the relationships within health care today in some parts of the country are so contentious that there is "no turning back" from the politics of destruction that lies ahead.

If all this book does is define the shape of the table at which all the relevant parties to a covenant can sit, and propose a paradigm and a vocabulary for the first discussion, it may be enough for now. To do more at this time would be to prematurely suppose an outcome that only a covenant can determine.

Why so many questions and so few answers?
Few health policy issues today have clear answers or easy resolutions, and I can't imagine that the next several decades will be any easier for those of us in this field. Today's health policy, which is so dominated by the economics of care, could benefit from an infusion of new ideas to frame our analyses. This is an offering of that type. I wanted to bring a new perspective, some structure for analysis, a vocabulary for negotiations and some tools to help.

Health care today could also benefit from an infusion of new questions. It is not only the answers to questions that are important, but the questions themselves. Some say, in fact, that the right question is more important than the right answer. Ancient wisdom says we can afford to be inefficient if we are working on the right question. Stephen Covey's work on effectiveness is built, in part, on a similar notion that it is not valuable to focus on how fast one can climb a ladder, if that ladder is leaning against the wrong tree.[2]

I applaud everyone in health care, e-commerce and telecommunications working to create efficiencies. Their work deserves support, encouragement and reward. Squeezing the cents from the dollars is a good thing. Squeezing the soul from the system is not. I'll continue to pose the questions that get to the soul of healing.

Will health care in the future be consumer-centric? Is covenant-centric going against the tide?
Health care of the near future will be consumer-centric. This is most likely a phase of our development as a society, and it may be a healthy transition. I hope that it will only be a phase and that we transition beyond it. Health care will benefit from consumers with the incentive to care for their health and the personal skills for doing so. Healers and communities can and should help them do that, and doing so may be the most important covenant-focused activity that healers and communities can fulfill in the near future. This consumer-centric attitude, however, should then transition towards interdependence among consumers, communities and healers. If health care of the future is only consumer-centered, lacking in covenants of obligation among the parties involved, the many challenges we face now will become serious problems, and the many opportunities before us today to solve problems won't be realized.

How can you expect that we can do what you advocate when all of our policy discussions are political debates? How can we get Congress involved?

We should talk to each other, not to Congress, about what ails us in health care. It is my observation that we turn to Congress reluctantly, and in anger, when the relationship between us breaks down, and we want the Congress to impose controls to fix the "other guy." I was in the audience at one of the farewell addresses of Congressman Barber Conable, at his departure to head the World Bank. "Do not expect us to lead," he announced. "We were elected to represent, not to lead. In that regard, we will have to be dragged kicking and screaming into any issue we deal with." Reluctant congressmen, dragged into issues after years of local-constituent anger and hostility, are not in the best frame of mind for crafting a health care future. Perhaps if we talked to each other, we could sort out our needs, our wants and our differences of opinion. This means that every encounter, every phone call and every e-mail becomes an opportunity to deal with someone else in the covenant. Take those opportunities. In those instances where Congress is already involved, let's at least advise them to avoid rash solutions and eleventh-hour compromises that please no one. Doing the first will take our time; doing the latter will require our restraint. Doing both is absolutely essential.

How can covenants help the uninsured in this country? Aren't doctors and managed care just shirking their responsibilities to make care available to them?

This is my favorite question. It may be my next book. It is such an immense topic that it deserves a book, or several! Some of the best minds in the country are struggling with this issue, and they have my respect. I hope they are prepared to fail, because, in my view, the current paradigm of health care financing provides them with few opportunities for success. Today, these policy and political leaders, along with healers, are confronting the challenge of retrofitting new, escalating, unrelenting demands into old laws, regulations and systems. It's a tight fit for a swelling foot in a worn-out shoe. The employer-based and tax-funded insurance systems have matured into no-fault financing systems precisely at the time when employment patterns changed, science produced cures and consumers aged and emerged as politically savvy, demanding change agents. My friends in the health care financing battles will make incremental changes, but they will not have the wherewithal for true reform unless the underlying relationships among the parties to the covenant engage each other first in the ways I have proposed.

In the meantime, it is my view that the healers in this country are already doing their part by providing a substantial amount of care to the uninsured. Whether they are physicians, nurses, institutions or pharmaceutical companies, their products and services are available for free and at reduced charges for those who cannot afford them. Even the healers in medical advertising provide free services to develop public health service messages. Providing care for those who cannot afford it is within the covenants that shape healing practices and, in my view, healers have done their part within the covenant.

It is time now to address similar covenant-focused questions to patients and communities. Should patients who can afford coverage but decline to get it be required to do so? Can patients who engage in high-risk lifestyles that drive up costs be required to change their behaviors? Should those who demand mandates be required to find funding sources in some other pocket than their own? Should every new mandate that increases the cost of coverage be matched with a patient- or community-focused responsibility that will create savings in some other part of the employer or managed care budget?

It seems more important to me, however, that the uninsured challenge us with questions about what we value in this country, how health care stacks up in that value equation and what kind of responsibility we feel to ourselves and to others as a result. It is clear to me that we value health and health care in this country. It is well that we should. I have seen health care systems on five other continents, and this one (even at its worst) is by far the best. We value health and health care above many other things in our lives, and we want everyone to enjoy its benefits as well. We value it so highly that we believe cost should never be a barrier to receiving care, and that when it is, it should be free—a gift, if you will. This is not a new idea. Health and healing have always been a gift, from the deity, as the early chapters in this book describe. Our attitudes are no different than those of our ancestors; our behaviors, however, are different. Inherent in the gift-giving of a covenant tradition is the proscription to be a giver as well as a receiver. In the ancient tradition, the Israelites received gifts as a part of their covenant and were then enjoined to preserve their own health, protect the health of others, and give to others in recognition of what they had received. Therein lies a message for all of us today.

Notes

Preface

[1]John H. Bryant and Zbigniew Bankowski, "Health Policy: Ethics and Human Values—An International Dialogue," XVIIIth Council for International Organizations of Medical Sciences (CIOMS), Switzerland: CIOMS, 1984.

Introduction

[1]Guenter Risse, *Mending Bodies, Saving Souls: A History of Hospitals,* New York: Oxford University Press, 1999, pp. 577–578.

[2]National Health Statistics Group, Office of the Actuary, "National health expenditures, 1996," *Health Care Financing Review,* 19(1) Health Care Financing Administration (HCFA) pub. No. 03400, Washington DC: U.S. Government Printing Office, fall, 1997.

[3]*Statistical Abstract of the United States: 1998* (118th edition), Washington, DC: U.S. Bureau of the Census, 1998, p. 129.

[4]Commonwealth Fund, *From Bench to Bedside: Preserving the Research Mission of Academic Health Centers: Findings and Recommendations of The Commonwealth Fund Task Force on Academic Health Centers,* New York: The Commonwealth Fund, April, 1999.

[5]Life expectancy at birth by race and sex: United States, 1940, 1950, 1960 and 1970–1995. U.S. National Center for Health Statistics, "Monthly Vital Statistics Report," *Vital Statistics of the United States,* Vol. 45, No. 11(S)2, June 12, 1997. Also at http://www.cdc.gov/nchswww/data/mv4511s2.pdf. Accessed July 1, 1999.

[6]"The gerontocrats," *Economist,* May 13, 1995, p. 32.

[7]http://www.aarp.org. Accessed February 15, 2000.

[8]National Health Statistics Group, Office of the Actuary, "National health expenditures, 1996," *Health Care Financing Review,* 19(1), Health Care Financing Administration (HCFA) pub. No. 03400, Washington, DC: U.S. Government Printing Office, fall 1997.

[9]"Comparing health care," *Fortune,* July 27, 1992, p. 80.

[10]Institute for the Future, Robert Wood Johnson Foundation, "Health and Health Care 2010." Available at http://www.rwjf.org/iftf. Accessed February 25, 2000.

[11]Projections concerning health care expenditures are updated routinely by the Congressional Budget Office. Available at http://www.cbo.gov. Accessed November 17, 1999.

[12]David Emmons and Gregory Wozniak, "Physician contractual arrangements with managed care organizations," *Socioeconomic Characteristics of Medical Practice,* Chicago, IL: American Medical Association, 1997.

[13]"What the doctor ordered," *Time,* 1952, 60(7):38–44.

[14]Charles Morris, "The health-care economy is nothing to fear," *Atlantic Monthly,* December, 1999, pp. 86–96.

Chapter 1

[1]W.F. Buckley, Jr., "Mr. Goodwin's great society," *National Review,* 1965, 17(36):760.
[2]David B. Morris, *The Culture of Pain,* Berkeley: University of California Press, 1991, p. 44.
[3]Lakshmi Raman and Gerald A. Winer, Evidence of Immanent Justice Reasoning in Adults. Paper presented at the 107th Annual American Psychological Association Convention, Boston, 1999.

Chapter 2

[1]S. Rushworth, *Sam Woods, American Healing,* Barrytown, NY: Station Hill Press, 1992, p. 35.
[2]Steven H. Gifis, *Barron's Law Dictionary,* Woodbury, NY: Barron's Educational, 1975, p. 49.
[3]William F. May, *The Physician's Covenant: Images of the Healer in Medical Ethics,* Philadelphia, PA: Westminster Press, 1983, p. 119.
[4]May, p. 108.
[5]Charles G. Cumston, *An Introduction to the History of Medicine,* London: Dawsons of Pall Mall, 1968, pp. 86–87.
[6]Irving I. Edgar, *The Origins of the Healing Art: A Psycho-Evolutionary Approach to the History of Medicine,* New York: Philosophical Library, 1978, p. 138.
[7]Edgar, pp. 135–138.
[8]Indiana University School of Medicine, 1997–1998 Student Manual. Available at http://www.medlib.iupui.edu/osca/smoath.htm. Accessed April 3, 2000.
[9]"Islamic Code of Medical Ethics, Declaration of Kuwait," adopted by the International Conference on Islamic Medicine, 1981. Available at http://www.phrusa.org/research/medicsoath.htm. Accessed October 31, 1999.
[10]J.A. Benson, Contemporary Use of Oaths and Covenants. Paper presented at the Institute of Medicine, Washington, DC, October 13, 1998.
[11]Gifis, p. 44.
[12]Gifis, p. 45.
[13]Gifis, p. 45.
[14]Donald Berwick, Janeway, P. Hiatt and R. Smith, "An ethical code for everybody in health care," *Brit Med J,* 1997, 15:1633–1634.
[15]Frank J. Molnar et al., "Assess the quality of newspaper medical advice columns for elderly readers," *California Medical Association Journal,* 1999; 161:393–395.
[16]Eli Ginzberg, "Ten encounters with the U.S. health sector, 1930–1999," *JAMA,* 1999; 282:1665–1668.
[17]Elia Kacapyr, "What's wrong with this picture?," *American Demographics,* September, 1998, pp. 18–19.
[18]*In The Physician's Covenant: Images of the Healer in Medical Ethics,* Philadelphia, PA: Westminster Press, 1983. William May describes the model of the physician-patient relationship in parent-child terms.

Chapter 3

[1]A. Etzioni, The Responsive Community: A Communitarian Perspective (Presidential Address, American Sociological Association, August 20, 1995), *Amer Sociological Rev,* February, 1996, pp. 1–11.
[2]A.D. Speigel, "Hammurabi's managed health care: Circa 1700 BC," *Managed Care,* May, 1997. Available at http://www.managedcaremag.com/archiveMC/9705/9705.hammurabi.shtml. Accessed November 29, 1998.

[3]Rates of noncompliance for epilepsy range from 30%–50% [I.E. Leppik, "How to get patients with epilepsy to take their medication: The problem of noncompliance," *Postgrad Med*, 1990, 88:253–256]; for arthritis from 55%–71% [W. van Elmeren and B. Horisberger, eds., *Socioeconomic Evaluation of Drug Therapy*, New York, NY: Springer-Verlag, 1998]; for hypertension to 40% [L.T. Clark, "Improving compliance and increasing control of hypertension: Needs of special hypertensive population," *Amer Heart J*, 1991:664–669]; and for diabetes from 40%–50% [M. Nagasawa, M.C. Smith and J.H. Barnes, "Meta-analysis of correlates of diabetes patients' compliance with prescribed medications," *The Diabetes Educator*, 1989, 16(3):192–200]. Even organ transplant patients, for whom medications prevent organ rejection and death, have noncompliance rates of near 20% [M. Rovelli, D. Palmeri, E. Vossler, S. Bartus, D. Hull and R. Schweitzer, "Noncompliance in organ transplant recipients," *Transplantation Proceedings*, 1989; 21:833–834]. The cost in terms of additional doctor visits is high. Excess hospital admissions are placed at $25 billion per year, nursing home admissions at $5 billion and lost productivity in the workplace at $50 billion [Task Force for Compliance, "Noncompliance with Medications: An Economic Tragedy with Important Implications for Health Care Reform," November, 1993, revised April, 1994. For further information, contact John Hawks, Task Force Executive Director, 2300 N. Charles Street, Suite 200, Baltimore, MD 21218, phone: 410-467-1100]. Even an aggressive intervention program using pharmacists to improve compliance for lipid-lowering agents, the compliance rates rose only to 84%. That increase is better than most programs, but is still not good enough if we are to achieve the cost-management goals that the public and payers have set for health care [B.M. Bluml, J.M. McKenney, M.J. Cziraky and R.K. Elswick, "Interim report for Project ImPACT: Hyperlipidemia," *J Amer Pharm Assoc*, 38(5):529–534].

[4]J.M. McGinnis and W.H. Foege, "Actual causes of death in the United States," *JAMA*, 1993, 270(18):2207–2212.

[5]C.L. Murray and A.D. Lopes, "Alternative projections of mortality and disability by cause 1990–2020: Global burden of disease study," *Lancet*, 1997, 349:1498–1504.

[6]N. Pronk, M. Goodman, P. O'Connor and B. Martinson, "Relationship between modifiable health risks and short-term health care charges," *JAMA*, 1999, 282(23):2235–2239.

[7]Centers for Disease Control and Prevention, "Tobacco Use—United States, 1900–1999," *JAMA*, 282(23):2202–2204.

[8]Lewin Group, "Costs of Obesity," for the American Obesity Association, Obesity Conference, Washington, DC, September 15, 1999.

[9]Healthy People 2000 Progress Review, Centers for Disease Control and Prevention, last updated on December 15, 1999. Available at http:/www.odphp.pdophs.dhhs.gove/pubs/hp2000. Accessed February 4, 2000.

[10]An entire issue of the *Journal of the American Medical Association* was devoted to obesity, edited by Richard M. Glass, M.D. and Phil B. Fontararosa, M.D., *JAMA*, 1999, 282(16):1493–1588.

[11]"Inside the industry—Obesity drugs: Drugmakers vie for market share," *American Health Line*, November 5, 1998.

[12]H. Taylor, Public Health, *The Harris Poll #60*, October 20, 1999.

[13]P.S. Mead, L. Slutskey, V. Dietz, L. McCaid, J. Bresee, C. Shapiro, P. Griffin and R. Tauxe, "Food-related illness and death in the United States," *Emerging Infectious Diseases*, 1999, 5(5). Available at http://www.edc.gov/mcidod/EID/vol5no5/mead.htm. Accessed September 18, 1999.

[14]Centers for Disease Control and Prevention, "Current trends in childhood lead poisoning—United States: Report to the Congress by the Agency for Toxic

Substances and Disease Registry," *MMWR*, 1988, 37(32):481–485. See also, "About Lead Poisoning," Alliance to End Childhood Lead Poisoning. Available at http://www.aeclp.org.

[15]J. Steinhauer, "Plan to fight West Nile Virus outlined," *New York Times*, December 17, 1999, p. B3.

[16]Personal communication with Robert Howard, Special Assistant for Media Relations, Center for Infectious Diseases, Centers for Disease Control and Prevention.

[17]Air Pollution and Respiratory Health, National Center for Environmental Health, Centers for Disease Control and Prevention. Available at http://www.cdc.gov/nceh/publicatns/1994/cdc/brosures/aripollu.htm. Accessed February 21, 2000.

[18]Teen Pregnancy, National Center for Chronic Disease Prevention and Health Promotion, Centers for Disease Control and Prevention. Available at http://www.cdc.gov/needphp/teen/html. Accessed August 16, 1999.

[19]Fetal Alcohol Syndrome, Division of Child Development, Disability and Health, Centers for Disease Control and Prevention. Available at http://www.cdc.gov/nceh/programs/cddh/fashome.htm. Accessed August 20, 1999.

[20]D.P. Rice, E.J. MacKenzie, A.S. Jones, S.R. Kaufman, G.V. DeLissovoy, W. Max, E. McLaughlin, T.R. Miller, L.S. Robertson, D.S. Salkever and G.S. Smith, *Cost of Injury in the United States*, Baltimore, MD: The John Hopkins University Press, 1989.

[21]T.R. Miller, M.N. Pindus, J.B. Douglass and S.B. Rossman, *Databook on Nonfatal Injury: Incidence, Costs and Consequences*, Washington, DC: Urban Institute Press, 1995.

[22]National Highway Traffic Safety Administration (NHTSA), *Promoting Safe Passage into the 21st Century*, Washington, DC: NHTSA, 1999.

[23]NHTSA, *National occupant protection use survey–1996, Research Note*, Washington, DC: NHTSA, 1997.

[24]P.J. Cook, B.A. Lawrence, J. Ludwig and T.R. Miller, "The medical costs of gunshot injuries in the United States," *JAMA*, 1999, (282):447–454.

[25]Unintentional Injury, National Center for Injury Prevention and Control, Centers for Disease Control and Prevention. Available at http://www.cdc.gov/ncipc. Accessed November 12, 1999.

Chapter 4

[1]Jayne Mackta, "The case for communication," *Lab Animal*, February, 2000, 29(2):38–40.

[2]Purnell Chopin, "Report from the president," *Howard Hughes Medical Institute Bulletin*, December, 1998. Available at http://www.hhmi.org/annual98/report/index.html. Accessed December 23, 1999.

[3]Lawrence Goldstein, "Investing in tomorrow's health care today," *Howard Hughes Medical Institute Bulletin*, February, 1996. Available at http://www.hhmi.org/communic/bulletin/Feb98/invest.htm. Accessed December 23, 1999.

[4]L. Goldstein. Available at http://www.hhmi.org/communic/bulletin/Feb98/invest.htm. Accessed December 23, 1999.

[5]Pharmaceutical Research and Manufacturers of America, *1999 Industry Profile*, Washington, DC: PhRMA, 1999, p. 13.

[6]Information available at http://www.AMProgress.org. Accessed February 11, 2000. Other activist activity at the University of Minnesota can be found in: Will Woodward, "On campus, animal rights vs. animal researchers: University of Minnesota emerges as a focal point," *Washington Post*, November 5, 1999, p. A01.

[7]Meridith Wadman, "U.S. Senate gets tough on animal activists," *Nature,* June 3, 1999, p. 397.

[8]Agriculture Fact Book, U.S. Department of Agriculture, Office of Communications, 1996.

[9]Katie McCabe, "Who will live and who will die?" *The Washingtonian,* August 1986, p. 114.

[10]Cited in Martin S. Pernick, *A Calculus of Suffering: Pain, Professionalism and Anesthesia in Nineteenth-Century America,* New York: Columbia University Press, 1985, p. 156.

[11]Viki D. Thompson Wylder, *Judy Chicago: Trials and Tributes,* Tallahassee, Florida: Florida State University Museum of Fine Arts, 1999.

[12]John G. Hubbell, "The 'animal rights' war on medicine," *Reader's Digest,* June, 1990, pp. 70–76.

[13]Personal Communication, HSUS Office of Membership.

[14]Report of confidential interviews, cited in New Jersey Association for Biomedical Research, The HSUS 2020 Initiative and Animal Rights, Strategic Health Policy International, 1999.

[15]The total amount of funds dedicated to identifying alternatives to the use of animals in research has not been tallied, but is estimated to be well over $7 million annually. Funds are provided by both public and private sector sources, including the National Institutes of Health, the National Toxicology Program, the Johns Hopkins Center for Alternatives to Animals in Testing, Proctor & Gamble, and the Alternatives Research and Development Foundation. Personal communication with Joanne Zurlow, Ph.D., Associate Director, Center for Alternatives to Animals in Testing.

Chapter 5

[1]The National Center for Health Services Research Agency was created nearly 25 years ago. The agency has since been renamed, it is now known as the Agency for Healthcare Research and Quality (AHRQ) and has a fiscal year 2000 budget of $107.05 million. This is not the only federal agency that conducts or funds this type of research. The Health Care Financing Administration, the Centers for Disease Control and Prevention, the Department of Defense, the Veterans Administration, and the Health Resources and Services Administration also conduct research to understand the delivery of health care.

[2]California Health Care Association, National Survey: Confidentiality of Medical Records, January 29, 1999. Available at http://www.chcf.org. Accessed October 12, 1999.

[3]Robert O'Harrow, Jr., "Prescription sales: Privacy fears," *Washington Post,* February 15, 1998, PA1, A18–19.

[4]The defendants in this case include CVS Pharmacy, Inc., Elensys Care Service, Inc., GlaxoWellcome, Inc., Warner-Lambert Company, Merck & Co., Inc., Biotech, Inc., Biogen, Inc., and Hoffman-LaRoche, Inc. Commonwealth of Massachusetts, Superior Court Department of the Trial Court, Civil Action No. 9800897-F.

[5]The exact number of comments will not be known until the comment period closes and the Department of Health and Human Services has the opportunity to review and tally them. Even without the variety of comments concerning the draft regulations, there are differences of opinion on the best ways to preserve privacy and most of those variations are at the state level. Of the five major bills introduced in the 105th Congress, the only major differences among these bills lie in how the federal standard would affect the flexibility of state laws. In the absence of feder-

al law, the states have acted to set standards of their own. Prior to 1999, only seven states had set regulations concerning how insurers could use medical records. Twenty-eight states included in their legislation the duty for physicians, insurers, health care institutions and other providers to maintain the confidentiality of computerized medical records. Concerning the penalties for unauthorized disclosure, seventeen states established civil penalties, nine states have criminal penalties and five states have both types of penalties. The remaining nineteen states established neither criminal nor civil penalties for unauthorized disclosure of medical records.

[6]Charles Greene Cumston, An Introduction to the History of Medicine, London, Dawsons of Pall Mall, 1968, pp. 86–87.

[7]Health Care Information Privacy, Louis Harris and Associates poll conducted for Equifax, 1993.

[8]Steven Jacobsen, Zhisen Xia, Mary Campion et al., "Potential effect of authorization bias on medical record research," Mayo Clin Prac, 1999, 74:330–338.

[9]Victor G. Freeman, Saif S. Rathore, Kevin P. Weinfurt, Kevin A. Schulman and Daniel P. Sulmasy, "Lying for patients: Physician deception of third-party payers," Arch Intern Med, 1999, 159:2263–2270.

[10]Max Frankel, "Snoops or germs?," New York Times Magazine, September 13, 1998, p. 44.

Chapter 6

[1]Oskar Kraus, Albert Schweitzer: His Work and His Philosophy, London: Adam & Charles Black, 1944, p. 26.

[2]Stuart Grossman et al., "Correlation of patient and caregiver ratings of cancer pain," J Pain and Symptom Manage, 1991, 6(2):53–57; Jamie H. Von Roenn et al., "Physician attitudes and practice in cancer pain management," Ann Intern Med, 1993, 119(2):121–126.

[3]National Pain Survey, Conducted for Ortho-McNeil Pharmaceutical, 1999; "Acute pain management: Operative or medical procedures and trauma," Clinical Practice Guideline No. 1, AHCPR Publication No. 92-0032, Rockville, MD: Agency for Health Care Policy and Research, Department of Health and Human Services, February, 1992.

[4]Clermont E. Dionne, "Low back pain," in Iain Crombie, Peter Croft, Steven Linton, Linda LeResche, and Michael Von Korff (eds.), Epidemiology of Pain, Seattle, WA: International Association for the Study of Pain, 1999, pp. 283–297.

[5]Reva C. Lawrence et al., "Estimates of the prevalence of arthritis and selected musculoskeletal disorders in the United States," Arthritis and Rheum, 1998, 41(5):778–799.

[6]Marilyn Marchione, "Headaches: Common, painful and expensive," Scripps Howard News Service, November 23, 1999.

[7]Pain and Absenteeism in the Workplace, Study conducted for Ortho-McNeil Pharmaceutical, 1997; International Pain Survey, conducted for Ortho-McNeil Pharmaceutical, 1999.

[8]The NIH Guide: New Directions in Pain Research I, Washington, DC: Government Printing Office, 1998.

[9]International Association for the Study of Pain, Subcommittee on Taxonomy, "Part II: Pain terms: A current list with definitions and notes on usage," Pain, 1979, 6:249–252.

[10]E.J. Cassell, The Nature of Suffering and the Goals of Medicine, New York: Oxford University Press, 1991, p. 36.

[11]National Hospice Organization (NHO), 1700 Diagonal Road, Suite 300,

Alexandria, VA 22314. Available at http://www.nho.org. Accessed October 15, 1999.

[12]C.S. Hill, "The negative influence of licensing and disciplinary boards and drug enforcement agencies on pain treatment with opioid analgesics," *J Pharm Care, Pain and Symptom Control,* 1993, 1:43–62; R. Nowak, "Cops and doctors: Drug busts hamper pain therapy," *J NIH Res,* 1980, 4:27–28.

[13]National Hospice Organization (NHO), 1700 Diagonal Road, Suite 300, Alexandria, VA 22314. Available at http://www.nho.org. Accessed October 15, 1999.

[14]J. Porter, and H. Jick, "Addiction rate in patients treated with narcotics," *New Engl J Med,* 1980, 302:123; R.K. Portnoy, and K.M. Foley, "Chronic use of opioid analgesics in non-malignant pain: Report of 38 cases," *Pain,* 1986, 25:171–186; E.M. Marks, and E.J. Sashar, "Undertreatment of medical inpatients with narcotic analgesics," *Ann Intern Med,* 1973, 78:173–181.

[15]According to the joint statement of the American Academy of Pain Medicine and the American Pain Society, physicians need not fear respiratory depression and other side effects of pain medicines, which are rare and can be managed with diet and other medical supports. Sedation and nausea are early side effects that usually dissipate with continued use of the medication, 1998.

[16]E. Emanuel, "Euthanasia and physician-assisted suicide: Attitudes and experiences of oncology patients," *Lancet,* 1996, 347(9018):1805; K.M. Foley, "The relationship of pain and symptom management to patient request for physician-assisted suicide," *J Pain and Symptom Manage,* 1991, 6:289–297.

[17]Richard Schulz, and Scott R. Beach, "Caregiving as a risk factor for mortality: The caregiver health effects study," *JAMA,* 1999, 282(23):2215–2219.

[18]Family Caregivers Association, 10400 Connecticut Ave., Kensington, MD, 20895-3994. Available at http://www.nfcacares.org. Accessed December 3, 1999.

[19]Joint Statement of the American Pain Society and the American Academy of Pain Management, 1998.

[20]Alabama, Alaska, Arizona, Arkansas, California, Colorado, Florida, Georgia, Iowa, Kansas, Louisiana, Massachusetts, Maryland, Minnesota, Missouri, Montana, Nebraska, Nevada, New Jersey, New Mexico, North Dakota, Ohio, Oklahoma, Oregon, Pennsylvania, Rhode Island, Tennessee, Texas, Utah, Vermont, Virginia, Washington, West Virginia, Wisconsin, Wyoming.

[21]Iowa, Rhode Island, South Dakota, Virginia, Oklahoma, South Carolina, Virginia, West Virginia, Arkansas and Maryland.

[22]Alabama, Arkansas, Illinois, Kansas, Maryland, Missouri, Vermont (some of these measures strengthen the language of earlier legislation).

[23]The American Academy of Pain Medicine, The American Pain Society, The Federation of State Medical Boards of the U.S., The Medical Board of California, The National Academy of Sciences, Institute of Medicine, The National Conference of Commissioners on Uniform State Laws, The National Conference of State Legislatures, The State Cancer Pain Initiatives.

[24]Joel B. Obermeyer, "Doctors urged to treat pain," *News and Observer* (Raleigh, NC), October 26, 1999.

[25]William T. McGivney and Glenna M. Crooks, "The care of patients with severe chronic pain in terminal illness," *JAMA,* 1984, 251(9):1181–1188.

Chapter 7

[1]Information at http://www.drini.com/mothertheresa/own_words/. Accessed March 18, 2000.

[2]Lawrence Altman, "U.N. issues grim report on the 11 million children orphaned

by AIDS," *New York Times,* December 2, 1999, p. A12. See also United Nations Press Release PI/1205, World AIDS Day held at headquarters, Focus on children orphaned by AIDS, December 1, 1999.

[3] Marilyn Chase, "New, virulent forms of tuberculosis spur concerns world-wide," *Wall Street Journal,* December 17, 1999, p. B1.

[4] David Satcher, "Tuberculosis—Battling an ancient scourge," *JAMA,* 1999, 282(21):1996.

[5] Judith Miller, "Study says new TB strains need an intensive strategy," *New York Times,* October 28, 1999, p. A6.

[6] Information available at http://www.worldbank.org. Accessed December 14, 1999.

[7] "Corporate hospitality," *Economist,* November 27, 1999, p. 71.

[8] Information available at http://www.gatesfoundation.org. Accessed December 14, 1999.

[9] Information available at http://www.capitalresearch.org. Accessed December 14, 1999.

[10] Information available at http://www.rotary.org. Accessed December 14, 1999.

[11] Information available at http://www.gatesfoundation.org. Accessed December 14, 1999.

[12] Information available at http://www.fdncenter.org. Accessed December 14, 1999.

[13] Gro Harlem Brundtland, International Trade Agreements and Public Health: WHO's Role, presented by video at the Conference on Increasing Access to Essential Drugs in Globalized Economy, Amsterdam, November 25–26, 1999.

[14] Lilly rushes antibiotic aid to more than one million Rwandan refugees, Lilly Press Release, July 27, 1994.

[15] "Lilly speeds needed drugs to Rwandan refugees," *FDA Today,* October 1994, pp. 4–5.

[16] "The goodwill pill mess," *Time,* 1996, 147(18):64.

[17] J.L. Zeballos, Health aspects of the Mexico earthquake—19 September, 1985," *Disasters,* 1986, 10:141–149.

[18] P. Autier, M.C. Ferir and A. Hairapetiien, "Drug supply in the aftermath of the 1988 Armenian earthquake," *Lancet,* 1990; 335:1388–1390.

[19] H.M. Ali, M.M. Homeida and M.A. Abdeen, "'Drug Dumping' in donations to the Sudan" (letter), *Lancet,* 1990, 336:745.

[20] L. Offerhaus, "Russia: Emergency drug goes awry," *Lancet,* 1990, 339:607.

[21] Personal communication, Hans Hogerziel, World Health Organization.

[22] Frank Greve, "Drug donations: A bitter pill?," *Philadelphia Inquirer,* June 16, 1999, p. 1.

[23] Department of Essential Drugs and Other Medicines, Guidelines for Drug Donations, World Health Organization, Geneva, 1999.

[24] Patrick Berckmans, Veronique Dawans, Gerard Schmets, Daniel Vandenbergh and Philippe Autier, "Inappropriate drug-donation practices in Bosnia and Herzegovina, 1992 to 1996," *New Engl J Med,* 337(25):1842–1845.

[25] Jacqueline Rieschick, "Drug donors get deductions for not-so-charitable contributions," *Tax Notes International,* January 13, 1999, 16:174–176.

[26] The Partnership for Quality Medical Donations (PQMD) is an alliance of pharmaceutical companies and private voluntary organizations working to improve the quality of medicine donations around the world. Their activities have been significant in representing the interests of their membership in continuing to donate medical products. Further information is available at http://www.pqmd.org.

[27] Personal communication, Sister Maura O'Donohue, M.D., Catholic Medical Mission Board.

[28]"Charitable giving: Will Americans be generous in the '90s?" *CQ Researcher,* 1993, 3(42):985–1008.

[29]Information available at http://www.merck.com. Accessed December 27, 1999.

[30]Information available at http://www.sb.com. Accessed December 27, 1999.

[31]Information available at http://www.glaxowellcome.com. Accessed December 27, 1999.

[32]Information available at http://www.iclinic.co.za/sept99/healthaid3.htm. Accessed December 29, 1999.

[33]Michael R. Reich, ed., *An Assessment of U.S. Pharmaceutical Donations: Players, Processes and Products,* Boston: Harvard School of Public Health, 1999.

[34]"Corporate hospitality," *Economist,* November 17, 1999, p. 71.

Chapter 8

[1]Patch Adams, *Gesundheit! Bringing Good Health to You, the Medical System, and Society Through Physician Service, Complementary Therapies, Humor, and Joy,* Rochester, Vermont: Healing Arts Press, 1993, p. 51.

[2]In instances where there are no citations concerning the individual mentioned, it is because the biographical sketches are drawn from my experiences with the individuals.

[3]E. Ransdell, "This 'killer app' saves money and lives," *Fast Company,* November 1999, pp. 112–113. See also www.diabeteswell.com.

[4]D. H. Freedman, "Intensive care," *Inc.,* February, 1999, pp. 72–80. See also http://www.griffinhealth.org.

[5]http://www.cvs.com.

[6]U. E. Reinhardt, "Medicare can turn anyone into a crook," *Wall Street Journal,* January 21, 2000, p. A18.

[7]J. Scott, G. Gade, M. McKenzie and I. Venohr, "Cooperative health care clinics: A group approach to individual care," *Geriatrics,* 1998, 53(3):86–81. See also J. Scott and B.J. Robertson, "Kaiser Colorado's Cooperative Health Care Clinic: A group approach to patient care," *Managed Care Quart,* 1996, 4(3): 41–45; A. Beck, J. Scott, P. Williams, B. Robertson, D. Jackson, G. Glade and P. Cowan, "A randomized trial of group outpatient visits for chronically ill older HMO members: The Cooperative Health Care Clinic," *J Amer Geriatr Soc,* 1997, 45(5):534–549.

[8]Center for Studying Health System Change, *Local Innovations Provide Managed Care for the Uninsured, Issue Brief Findings from HSC,* Mathematica Policy Research, no. 25, January, 2000.

[9]H. D. Scott, J. Bell, S. Geller and M. Thomas, "Physicians helping the underserved: The Reach Out Program, *JAMA,* 2000, 283(1):99–104.

[10]"The Nursing Center in Concept and Practice: Delivery and Financing Issues in Serving Vulnerable People," National Health Policy Forum Issue Brief No. 746, September 13, 1999.

[11]Personal communications with Brian Robinson, ParExcel and Rima Cohen, Greater New York Hospital Association.

[12]A. Sharpe, "Health care: Discounted fees cure headaches, some doctors find," *Wall Street Journal,* September 15, 1998, B1. See also http://www.simplecare.com.

[13]*Healthy People in Healthy Communities, A Dialogue Guide,* Chicago, IL: The Coalition for Healthier Cities and Communities, 1999. See also *Transforming Health Care: Lessons from Community Partnerships,* National Community Care Network Demonstration Program, Chicago, IL: Health Research and Education Trust, 1999; and C.F. Adams (ed.), *Voices from America: Ten Healthy Community Stories from across the Nation,* Chicago, IL: Coalition for Healthier Cities and Communities and the Health Research and Educational Trust, 1998.

[14]*What creates health? Individuals and communities respond, a national study conducted by DYG, Inc. for the Healthcare Forum,* San Francisco, 1994. This study was conducted in partnership with the W. K. Kellogg Foundation, the Healthcare Forum, the Healthier Communities Partnership and the National Civic League (single copies are available free by calling 415-356-4317); See also *Leadership for a Healthy 21st Century,* Chicago, IL: The American Hospital Association, 1999 (single copies are available at no charge by calling 1-800-AHA-2626).

[15]D. Cummings, T. Hamilton, B. Crawford and B. Cherney, Integrating Education, Technology, Wellness and Community with Traditional Medicine: A View of the Future. Paper presented at the Ninth National CEO Summit, Atlanta, March 29–30, 1999.

[16]Information concerning Celebration Health is based on personal communications with Des Cummings, Florida Hospital Health Systems.

[17]Information concerning the ACT Project is based on personal communications with Brian Crawford, Center for Health Futures at Celebration Health; Kathryn Johnson, Wynne Grossman and Michael Bilton of the Health Forum; and Robert Gold, Macro International.

[18]Outcomes Toolkit: The Results Oriented System for Community Improvement, Healthcare Forum of the American Hospital Association and Macro International. Further information is available by contacting the Health Forum Customer Service Department at 1-800-821-2039.

Chapter 9

[1]John H. Bryant, and Zbigniew Bankowski, *Health Policy, Ethics and Human Values—An International Dialogue,* XVIIIth Council for International Organizations of Medical Sciences (CIOMS), Switzerland: CIOMS, 1984, p. 7.

[2]D. Berwick, Janeway, P. Hiatt, and R. Smith, "An ethical code for everybody in healthcare." *Brit Med J,* 1997, 315:1633–1634.

[3]In one study of routine neonatal circumcision, 63% of parents did not discuss the procedure with any medical professional prior to admission to the hospital for childbirth and 20% were confronted with the decision at that time. Of those parents delivering male children, 37% discussed circumcision with a medical professional, 9% with friends, 20% with the hospital admissions clerk and 34% discussed it with no one. A.J. Herrera and J.B. Trouern-Trend, "Routine neonatal circumcision," *Am J Dis Child,* 1979, 133:1069–1070.

[4]Lynn Clothier, personal communication.

[5]J.A. Benson, Contemporary Use of Oaths and Covenants. Paper presented at the Institute of Medicine, Washington, DC, October 13, 1998.

[6]L. Foster, "The Johnson & Johnson Credo and the Tylenol Crisis," *New Jersey Bell Journal Reprint.* Copies of this reprint, as well as a copy of the Credo may be obtained through the Johnson & Johnson Corporate Communications Department at 732-524-0400.

[7]*Putting Patients First®: Patient Rights and Responsibilities,* Washington, DC: National Health Council, 1995.

[8]Martin Wasserman, M.D., personal communication.

Epilogue

[1]PMPM refers to per member per month and is the payment made to a plan or physician provider to care for the patients in the plan each month of the patient enrollment.

[2]S. Covey, *The 7 Habits of Highly Effective People: Restoring the Character Ethic,* New York, NY: Simon & Schuster, 1989.

Index

A

Accelerating Community
   Transformation (ACT), 165–166
   Outcomes Toolkit, 167–168
access
   to healers, 57–58
   to medicine, 127–128
accountability, 56–58
Act
   Animal Enterprises Protection
      Act, 80
   Animal Welfare Act, 87
   National Chimpanzee Research
      Retirement Act, 87
   Health Insurance Portability and
      Accountability Act of
      1996 (HIPAA), 99
ACT Community Outcomes Toolkit,
   167–168
Adams, Patch, 149–151
Agency for Health Care Research
   and Quality (AHRQ), 56
air pollution, cost, 66
alcohol, cost, 66
alternative medicine, 170–171
   expenditures, 49–50
American Academy of Pain
   Management, 115
American Association of Patients and
   Providers (AAPP), 160
American Medical Association, 4
American Pain Society, 115
anger, xvi
animal
   research. See animal research
   rights, 82–84, 89–92
   role, 83–85
animal activism
   objective, 90
   People for the Ethical Treatment
      of Animals (PETA), 80

public support, 86–88
   strategies, 85–86
Animal Enterprises Protection Act, 80
animal research, 77, 80–81, 89–92
   covenant in, 77–92
   debate, 79–85, 91–92,
      189–190
   defense, 88–89
   ethics, 82–83
Animal Welfare Act, 87
Asclepius, 11–12, 14
Associations
   American Association of Patients
      and Providers (AAPP), 160
   American Medical Association, 4
   National Association for
      Biomedical Research (NABR),
      88–89
AstraZeneca, 164

B

Bashe, Gil, 151–152
Bayer, 163
behavior, 63–65, 68, 69–70
Bergman, William, 116–117
Berwick, Donald, 37, 178
billing. See records
Buckley, William F. Jr., 3
Buddhism, 10

C

Celebration Health, 160–164
   and community, 164–166
change, time and, 174
Charmel, Pat, 153
Chicago, Judy, 84–85
children, research, 84
Christianity, 8, 12–14
clinics
   Cooperative Health Care Clinics
      (CHCC), 156–158

Clinton Administration, 4
comedy, as therapy, 7
communication
    and animal research, 88–89
    see also news media
community, 160–164, 171
    Accelerating Commmunity
        Transformation (ACT),
        165–166
    covenants, 46–48
    covenants of grant, 65–68
    and drug abuse, 119–120
    and healers, 160–168
    uninsured and, 158
Community Health Improvement
    Council (CHIC), 164
compassion, 120–121
Compassionate Pain Relief Bill,
    113–114
compensation, 55
compliance, 63
    see also behavior
comprehensive consumer satisfaction
    survey (CAHPS), 56
Conable, Barber, 193
confidentiality, 93–94, 101
    questions, 103–105
    see also privacy
Congress, 133–114, 118–119, 192
consent, 103–104
consumer
    comprehensive consumer
        satisfaction survey (CAHPS), 56
    consumer-centric health care,
        192
continuity, 173–174
contracts
    covenants vs. 26
    defined, 35
    emergence of, 34–37
Cooperative Health Care Clinics
    (CHCCs), 156–158
cost
    air pollution, 66
    alcohol, 66
    alternative medicine, 49–50
    behavior, 63–65
    burden, 67–68
    of health care, 57–58, 63,
        65–67, 102, 103
    hospitals, 58
    infectious disease, 65, 66
    influenza, 66

injuries, 66–67
    lifestyle, 64
    rabies, 65–66
    reduction, 94
    smoking, 64
    traffic accidents, 66–67
cost-effectiveness, 61
covenants, xvii–xviii, 1–2, 36,
    189–194
    and animal research, 77–92
    and communities, 46–48,
        160–168
    and compassion, 120–121
    and confidentiality, 93–94,
        102–103
    defined, 25
    and donations, 134–136,
        141–146
    effectiveness and efficiency vs.
        personal privacy and
        confidentiality tradeoffs,
        93–94, 102–103, 105–108
    efficiency of, 93–108
    emerging, 151–168
    evolution of, 185–186
    existing, 147
    formula for, 25
    and future, 168
    gifts in, 172–173
    healers, 39–44, 151–158
    and healing, 149–168
    Hippocrates, 29–30
    interdependence of, 48–51
    Maimonides, 29–32
    meaning 24–26
    modern, 36–39
    new, 39–44, 169–187
    origin of, 24–26
    and pain relief, 110–111,
        120–124
    patient-healer, 44–46
    in patients' rights 55–76
    and privacy, 93–108
    reciprocity in, 58–60, 70
    relationships in, 191
    tradition of, 23–51
    and uninsured, 158–160
    see also oaths
covenants of grant, 26–28, 34,
    182–183
    limitations of, 60–65
    limitations with communities in,
        65–68

covenants of obligation, 26, 28–29,
    30–31, 34, 170–171, 174–178
  with communities, 68–70
  conditions of, 175–178
  creating, 73–76, 178–180
  with patients, 68–70
  rationale in, 68–70
  statement of relationships,
    180–182
Crooks, Jim, 124
Crooks, Nancy, 124
Cummings, Des, 152–153
CVS, 98, 99, 153

D

data
  collection and use, 104
  Health Plan Employer Data and
    Information Set (HEDIS), 56
  management, 104
  uses, 106–107
  see also records
databases, 98
Davies, Robert, 143
Death with Dignity Act, 118
developing world, 125–146
diabetes, 152
Diagnosis-Related Group (DRG), 38
disease
  curing, 77–92
  food-related, 65
  history of, 6–7
Disney, 161
dissatisfaction, 59–60
divinity, 1, 5, 6–7, 9–10
donations, 127–146
  covenants and, 134–136,
    141–146
  drug, 128–130, 132–133
  Guidelines for Drug Donations,
    133–134
  Internal Revenue Service,
    136–137
  international, 131–133
  Notre Dame University, meeting,
    135–136, 141–142
  policy, 137–138
  quality of, 144
  unusable, 136
drug abuse, 119–120
  pain relief and, 112–113, 117
drug policy, 137

E

education, 99
effectiveness and efficiency vs.
    personal privacy and
    confidentiality tradeoffs, 93–94
  covenant and, 102–103,
    105–108
  details, 95–97, 103–105
  patients, 100–101
efficiency
  and covenants, 93–108
  data in, 95–97
Elensys, 98, 99
Eli Lilly, 128–130
emerging covenants, 151–168
Emmens, Matt, 152–153
encephalitis
  West Nile Virus (WNV)
    Encephalitis, 65
epidemiology, 68
Essential Drug List (EDL), 137–138
ethics, 25, 33
  animal research, 82–83
  Islamic Code of Medical Ethics,
    33
Etzioni, Amitai, 55
executives, oath, 40

F

fee, 57
fetal alcohol syndrom (FAS), 66
filariasis, 142
Foege, Bill, 155
funding
  development projects, 127
  uninsured, 158

G

General Electric, 163–164
Giant (pharmacy), 98, 99
gift, divine, 3–22
Ginzberg, Eli, 46
GlaxoWellcome, 98, 99, 163
government regulators, 145
grants, 78
Great Society, The, 3
Greece, 10, 12
Guidelines for Drug Donations,
    133–134, 138–139

H

Hammurabi, Code of, 55

head injury, cost, 67
healers and healing, xvi, 5, 14–16,
178–179
  and accountability for quality,
  56
  and accountability for access
  and cost, 57–58
  American public policy, 4
  and community, 125–146,
  160–168
  contemporary, 151–156
  within covenant tradition, 23–54
  covenants with patients 44–46,
  151–158
  divine gift, 3–22
  efficiency, 94, 95–97
  foundations, 1–2
  healer-community relationship,
  185
  healer-patient relationship,
  xvi–xviii, 185
  and health care, 149, 169–187
  holistic, 162–164
  and interdependence, 50–51
  and pain, 115–116
  secular traditions, 14–16
health care
  Agency for Health Care
  Research and Quality
  (AHRQ), 56
  challenges, 53–54
  and covenants, 189–194
  and global community,
  126–128
  government and, 3–4
  healing and, 147–148,
  169–187
  investments, 78
  Joint Commission on
  Accreditation of Healthcare
  Organizations (JCAHO), 115
  Maryland Department of Health
  and Mental Hygiene,
  184–185
  National Committee for Quality
  Assurance (NCQA), 56
  National Health Council,
  183–185
  opportunities, 53–54
  Reach Out: Physicians' Initiative
  to Expand Care to
  Underserved Americans,
  158–159

secular traditions, 14–16
  Social Health Index, 47–48
Health Insurance Portability and
  Accountability Act of 1996
  (HIPAA), 99
Health Insurance Training and
  Education (HITE) Network, 159
Health Plan Employer Data and
  Information Set (HEDIS), 56
herbs, 15–16, 18
Hilleman, Maurice R., 154
Hippocrates, 11–12, 29–30
Hippocratic Oath, 32–33, 34–35
  privacy and, 100
history, xvi–xviii, 1–2, 5–22, 55
Hittites, 25
HIV/AIDS, 887, 142, 155
  activists, 79
HMOs, 27–28
hospitals, and cost, 58
Humane Society of the United States
  (HSUS), 85–86, 87, 90

I

Indiana Health Centers, 180–181
illness, and pain, 109–110
industry, cooperation with, 142
infectious disease, cost of, 65, 66
influenza, cost of, 66
injuries, cost of, 66–67
Inlander, Charles B. "Charlie," 153
insurance, 51, 57, 59
  Health Insurance Training and
  Education (HITE) Network, 159
  see also uninsured
interdependence, 48–51, 55–76
international issues, 190
investments, in health care, 78
Islamic Code of Medical Ethics, 33

J

Jesus, 13
Johnson, Lyndon B., 3
Johnson & Johnson Company, 163
  credo, 182–183
Joint Commission on Accreditation of
  Healthcare Organizations
  (JCAHO), 115
Jones, Judy Miller, 153–154
Judaic law, 9–10
justice, immanent, 7–9

K

Kessler, David, 129
Kucinich, Dennis J., 136–137
Kydd, Ronald, 20–21

L

law, 5–6, 25–26
    contracts, 35–36
    divine, 9–10
    enforcement, 120
    and pain, 109–124
legislation, 118–119
    animal activism, 86–87
    pain relief, 113–114
    privacy, 100–101, 105
    see also Act
Lerner, Julie, 152
Lerner, Paul, 152
license, 16
lifestyle, 51, 161–162
    costs, 63–64
    see also behavior
litigation, 99, 116–117
    animal activism, 86–87
    privacy, 100–101

M

Maimonides, 30–32, 35
malaria, 142
malevolence, 7–9
Maryland Department of Health and
    Mental Hygiene, 184–185
May, William, 26, 28–29, 36,
    173–174
media. See news media
Medicaid, 3
Medicare, 3–4
medication, 127–128
    Essential Drug List, 137–138
    and global community,
        125–146
    pain relief, 112–113
medicine
    alternative, 170–171
    Christian, 12–14
    Hippocratic, 11–12
    mystery and, 19–21
    shamanic, 17–19
Meyers, Abbey, 153
Middle Ages, 13–16
miracle-focused healing, models,
    20–21

mischief, 7–9
models, emerging, 149–168
Mosaic Law, 9–10
Moses, covenant, 28
Muhammad, 12
mystery
    in Christian medicine, 12–14
    of health and disease, 6–7
    in Hippocratic medicine 11–12
    in modern medicine, 19–21
    in shamanic medicine, 17–19

N

National Association for Biomedical
    Research (NABR), 88–89
National Chimpanzee Research
    Retirement Act, 87
National Committee for Quality
    Assurance (NCQA), 56
National Health Council, 183–185
Native Americans, 18
New Age, 19–21
news media, 129, 171
    confidentiality, 97–98
    negative, 102
    see also communication; public
    relations
Nightingale Pledge, 40
Noah, covenant, 27
nurses, oath, 40
Nursing Center, 159

O

oaths, 32–34, 39–42, 105–106
obligation, 62
    needy patients, 137–141
    see also covenants of obligation;
    responsibility
O'Donohue, Maura, 155
Outcomes Toolkit, 167–168

P

pain, 109–124
    American Academy of Pain
        Management, 115
    American Pain Society, 115
    Compassionate Pain Relief Bill,
        113–114
    covenant and, 109–124
    healers and, 115–116
    heroin, 113–114

management vs. drug abuse,
117
relief, 112–115
research, 84
Pain Relief Promotion Act of 1999,
119
partnerships, 164
Pascale, Blasé, 8
patents, 137–138
patient, xvi, 171
patient-community relationship,
46–48, 186
patient-healer relationship,
44–46
rights and covenant, 55–76
Patients' Bill of Rights, 70–72
patients' rights, 70–73, 184
payers, 69
payment. See cost; insurance
pediatric research, 84
Peer Review Organizations (PROs),
56
Pellegrino, Edmund, 169
People for the Ethical Treatment of
Animals (PETA), 80
pharmacists, 153
oath, 39, 41
politics, xv, 193
practices, ancient, 10–11
prayer, 19–20, 21–22
Prendergast, Joe, 152
prevention, 60–61
see also vaccines
primates, 84, 87
see also animal research
privacy, 94, 97–99, 101–102
covenant, and, 102–103,
105–108
efficiency vs. 93–108
legislation, 100–101
questions, 103–105
violations, penalties, 105
see also confidentiality
private sector, 143
profit, 145
Protestant Reformation, 16
public health, xiv–xv, 43–44, 47,
65–68, 68–69
public policy, 107
public relations, disasters, 129–131
see also news media

rabies, cost, 65–66
Reach Out: Physicians' Initiative to
Expand Care to Underserved
Americans, 158–159
reciprocity, in covenant relationship,
58–60
records
billing data, 95–97
medical, 96
review and correction, 104–105
see also confidentiality; data
Reich, Michael, 142
Reinhardt, Uwe, 156
relief
agencies, 139–140
efforts, 128–133
research, 77–92
Agency for Health Care
Research and Quality
(AHRQ), 56
children, 84
debating, 79–80
National Association for
Biomedical Research (NABR),
88–89
results, 79
spending, 79
subjects, 81–82, 84
see also animal research
responsibility
community, 75
donations, 144
healer, 75
patient, 62–63, 72–73, 75
policymakers, 76
researchers, 90–91
roots, 55
retribution, 7–9
rights
covenant in patients' rights,
55–76
patients', 70–73, 184
Patients' Bill of Rights, 70–72
roots, 55
risk, 128
river blindness, 142
Rushworth, Stan, 23
Rwanda, 128–130

sacred, 23–24

history, 1, 5–6
and secular, 21–22
saints, 13–14, 15
Satan, 15–16
Schweitzer, Albert, 109
scientists, oath, 42–43
Scott, John, 156
secular, and sacred, 21–22
security, 101
questions, 103–105
self-interest, 35–36
Shalala, Donna E., 93
shaman, 9, 17–19
SimpleCare, 160
smallpox, 155
smoking, cost, 64
Social Health Index, 47–48
Stark, Fortney H. "Pete," 136–137
Strategic Health Policy
International, xv
strategies, in animal research, 85–86
suffering, 111–112, 116–118
easing, 112–113
see also pain
suicide, assisted, 118
survey
comprehensive consumer
satisfaction survey (CAHPS), 56

T

Taoism, 11
tax policy, U.S., 137, 140–141
teenage pregnancy, cost, 66
terminal illness, 14–15, 63
see also pain
texts, ancient, 10–11
Theresa, Mother, 125
traffic accidents, cost, 66–67
trust, 102
tuberculosis, 125–126
Tylenol®, poisonings, 183

U

uninsured, 158–160, 193–194

V

vaccines, 61, 127–128
Vagelos, P. Roy, 154
volunteers, 158–159, 178–179
von Bingen, Hildegard, 16

W

Wasserman, Martin, 184–185
West Nile Virus (WNV) Encephalitis,
65
wisdom, of divine law, 9–10
World Bank, 193
World Health Organization, 137,
143
drug donations, 133–134
World Trade Organization, 1999
meeting, 137–138

About the Author

Glenna M. Crooks, Ph.D., former Deputy Assistant Secretary for Health for the Reagan administration, is founder and president of Strategic Health Policy International, Inc. (SHPI). Based in Philadelphia, Pennsylvania and Washington, DC, SHPI assists businesses and governments to understand and manage policy and political issues in health care.

At SHPI, Dr. Crooks counsels government and business executives in negotiating the challenges of leadership in today's rocky health care environment. Dr. Crooks has participated in the health care arena for more than twenty years. After leaving the United States Department of Health and Human Services, she developed and managed global policy operations at Merck & Company, for domestic and international markets. There she rose to become Vice President for Worldwide Operations of Merck's vaccine business.

SHPI works with health products and services companies, health providers, venture firms, trade associations and governments in North America, Europe, Asia, Africa, and Latin America. SHPI provides a range of services from formulating health policy and political analyses to designing strategy and management; from moderating and chairing meetings and facilitating consensus to negotiating and resolving conflicts; from speaking on select topics to customizing topics for client needs; and from training and mentoring to coaching and briefing executives.

Dr. Crooks is on the Board of Directors of American Biogenetics, Inc. and is an Adjunct Professor of Health Policy at the University of the Sciences in Philadelphia. She is the recipient of numerous public and private sector awards, including the Surgeon General's Medallion, the highest award in public health, from Surgeon General C. Everett Koop.